An Illustrated Review of the URINARY SYSTEM

Glenn F. Bastian

HarperCollins CollegePublishers

Executive Editor: Bonnie Roesch
Cover Designer: Kay Petronio
Production Manager: Bob Cooper
Printer and Binder: Malloy Lithographing, Inc.
Cover Printer: The Lehigh Press, Inc.

AN ILLUSTRATED REVIEW OF THE URINARY SYSTEM

by Glenn F. Bastian

Copyright © 1994 HarperCollins College Publishers

Library of Congress Cataloging-in-Publication Data

Bastian, Glenn F.
        An illustrated review of the urinary system / Glenn F. Bastian.
            p.   cm. — (Illustrated review of anatomy and physiology ;1)
        ISBN 0-06-501711-0
        1. Urinary organs—Physiology—Outlines, syllabi, etc. 2. Urinary
    organs—Anatomy—Outlines, syllabi, etc. 3. Urinary organs—
    Atlases. I. Title. II. Title: Urinary System. III Series:
    Bastian, Glenn F.   Illustrated review of anatomy & physiology.
    QP248.B37   1994
    612.4'6—dc20   94-20230
                                                                CIP

94 95 96 9 8 7 6 5 4 3 2 1

CONTENTS

LIST OF TOPICS & ILLUSTRATIONS

Text: One page of text is devoted to each of the following topics. *Illustrations are listed in italics.*

PREFACE

An Illustrated Review of Anatomy and Physiology is a series of ten books written to help students effectively review the structure and function of the human body. Each book in the series is devoted to a different body system.

My objective in writing these books is to make very complex subjects accessible and nonthreatening by presenting material in manageable-size bits (one topic per page) with clear, simple illustrations to assist the many students who are primarily visual learners. Designed to supplement established texts, they may be used as a student aid to jog the memory, to quickly recall the essentials of each major topic, and to practice naming structures in preparation for exams.

INNOVATIVE FEATURES OF THE BOOK

(1) Each major topic is confined to one page of text.

A unique feature of this book is that each topic is confined to one page and the material is presented in outline form with the key terms in boldface or italic typeface. This makes it easy to scan quickly the major points of any given topic. The student can easily get an overview of the topic and then zero in on a particular point that needs clarification.

(2) Each page of text has an illustration on the facing page.

Because each page of text has its illustration on the facing page, there is no need to flip through the book looking for the illustration that is referred to in the text ("see Figure X on page xx"). The purpose of the illustration is to clarify a central idea discussed in the text. The images are simple and clear, the lines are bold, and the labels are in a large type. Each illustration deals with a well-defined concept, allowing for a more focused study.

PHYSIOLOGY TOPICS (1 text page : 1 illustration)
Each main topic in physiology is limited to one page of text with one supporting illustration on the facing page.

Anatomy Topics (1 text page : several illustrations)
For complex anatomical structures a good illustration is more valuable than words. So, for topics dealing with anatomy, there are often several illustrations for one text topic.

(3) Unlabeled illustrations have been included.
In Part II, all illustrations have been repeated without their labels. This allows a student to test his or her visual knowledge of the basic concepts.

(4) A Pronunciation Guide has been included.
Phonetic spellings of unfamiliar terms are listed in a separate section, unlike other textbooks where they are usually found in the glossary or spread throughout the text. The student may use this guide for pronunciation drill or as a quick review of basic vocabulary.

(5) A glossary has been included.
Most textbooks have glossaries that include terms for all of the systems of the body. It is convenient to have all of the key terms for one system in a single glossary.

ACKNOWLEDGMENTS

I would like to thank the reviewers of the manuscript for this book who carefully critiqued the text and illustrations for their effectiveness: William Kleinelp, Middlesex County College; Robert Smith, University of Missouri, St. Louis, and St. Louis Community College, Forest Park; and Pamela Monaco, Molloy College. Their help and advice are greatly appreciated. Kay Petronio is to be commended for her handsome cover design and Bob Cooper has my gratitude for keeping the production moving smoothly. Finally, I am greatly indebted to my editor, Bonnie Roesch, for her willingness to try a new idea, and for her support throughout this project. I invite students and instructors to send any comments and suggestions for enhancements or changes to this book to me, in care of HarperCollins, so that future editions can continue to meet your needs.

Glenn Bastian

1 Structures and Functions

STRUCTURES AND FUNCTIONS / Overview

DEFINITIONS

Renal   Pertaining to the kidney.

Nephron   A microscopic tubule, which is the basic functional and structural unit of the kidney. Each kidney contains about one million nephrons.

Nephrology   The scientific study of the kidney.

Urology   A branch of medicine that is concerned with the urinary tract in both males and females, and with the external reproductive organs (genitalia) in males.

STRUCTURES

The urinary system consists of two kidneys, two ureters, one urinary bladder, and one urethra.

(1) Kidneys   The paired kidneys are located in the lumbar region; they are about 5 inches long and are shaped like kidney beans.

(2) Ureters   Ureters are tubes that carry urine from the kidneys to the urinary bladder.

(3) Urinary Bladder   The urinary bladder is a hollow muscular organ. It stores about 800 ml of urine.

(4) Urethra   The urethra is a tube that carries urine from the urinary bladder out of the body. In the female it is about 1.5 inches long; in the male it is about 8 inches long and also functions as a duct through which semen is discharged during sexual intercourse.

KIDNEY FUNCTIONS

The principal function of the kidneys is homeostasis—the maintenance of a relatively stable internal environment (the extracellular fluid or ECF).

(1) Water and Electrolyte Balance   The kidneys regulate the water content, electrolyte (mineral ion) composition, and acidity of the body fluids.

(2) Removal of Wastes and Foreign Chemicals   The kidneys remove toxic nitrogenous waste products from the blood and excrete them in the urine; nitrogenous wastes are products of the catabolism of proteins, nucleic acids, and muscle creatine. The kidneys also remove foreign chemicals and certain antibiotics from the blood.

(3) Secretion of Hormones   The kidneys secrete or activate three hormones: erythropoietin, calcitriol, and angiotensin II. *Erythropoietin* is secreted by the kidneys; it stimulates the production of red blood cells in bone marrow. *Calcitriol* is activated in the kidneys; it stimulates the reabsorption of dietary calcium and phosphate from the GI tract. *Angiotensin II* is activated by a series of reactions that are triggered by renin, an enzyme secreted by the kidneys; it raises the blood pressure.

RENAL PROCESSES

Urine is formed as filtered blood plasma passes through nephrons. It involves three basic processes: glomerular filtration, tubular reabsorption, and tubular secretion.

(1) Glomerular Filtration   The movement of plasma from blood capillaries into nephrons.

(2) Tubular Reabsorption   The movement of useful substances (nutrients, ions, and water) from the fluid inside the nephrons back into the blood of nearby capillaries (peritubular capillaries).

(3) Tubular Secretion   The movement of substances from the blood in peritubular capillaries into the filtered fluid. Excess hydrogen, potassium, and ammonium ions enter the fluid in this way.

URINARY SYSTEM

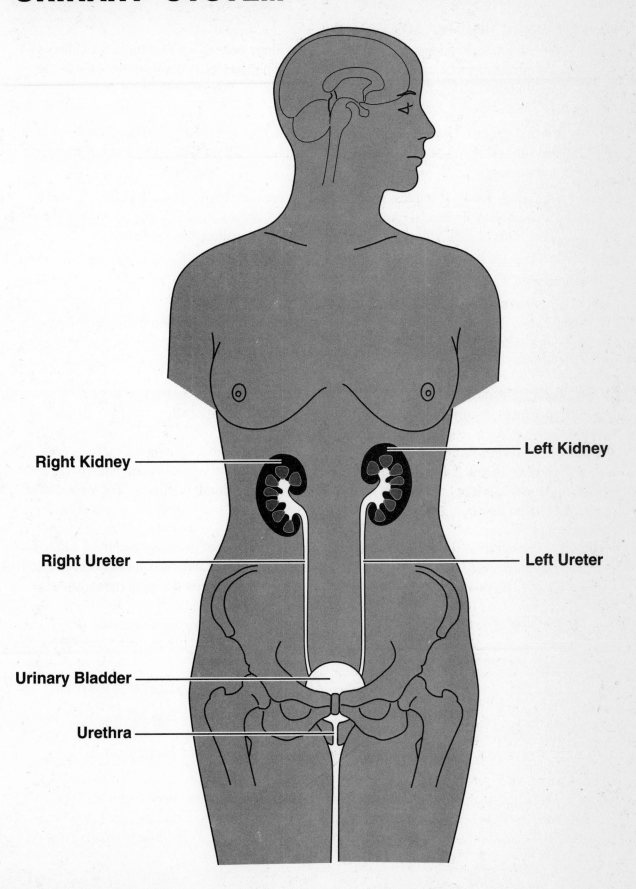

Right Kidney

Left Kidney

Right Ureter

Left Ureter

Urinary Bladder

Urethra

STRUCTURES AND FUNCTIONS / **Kidneys**

LOCATION, SIZE, AND SHAPE

The kidneys are a pair of reddish organs shaped like kidney beans. An average adult kidney is 4 to 5 inches long, 2 to 3 inches wide, and 1 inch thick. They are located above the waist in the posterior region of the abdominal cavity, between the levels of the 12th thoracic and 3rd lumbar vertebrae.

Retroperitoneal Organ   The kidneys are called retroperitoneal organs, because they are located behind the peritoneal lining of the abdomen (between the parietal peritoneum and the posterior wall of the abdomen).

Hilus   (also called *hilum*)   The hilus is a notch in the concave border of each kidney, where a ureter is attached. Blood vessels, lymphatic vessels, and nerves enter and exit the kidney through the hilus. The hilus of each kidney opens into a large cavity called the *renal sinus*.

STRUCTURES

Tissue Layers   Three layers of tissue surround each kidney.

Renal Capsule   The innermost layer. A smooth, transparent, fibrous membrane continuous with the outer coat of the ureter at the hilus.

Adipose Capsule   The middle layer. A mass of fatty tissue surrounding the renal capsule.

Renal Fascia   The outermost layer. A thin layer of dense irregular connective tissue that anchors the kidney to its surrounding structures and to the abdominal wall.

Medulla   The inner region of a kidney is called the medulla.

Renal Pyramid   The medulla consists of 8 – 18 cone-shaped structures called renal pyramids. The tip (or apex) of a renal pyramid is called a *renal papilla* (plural: papillae). The wide end of the cone is called the *base*.

Cortex   The cortex is the outer reddish area visible in a coronal (frontal) section of a kidney. It extends from the *renal capsule* to the bases of the pyramids and into the spaces between them.

Renal Column   Renal columns are the regions of the cortex between the renal pyramids.

Renal Pelvis   The hilus of each kidney opens into a large cavity called the *renal sinus*. Inside the renal sinus, a funnel-shaped cavity called the renal pelvis collects urine from nephrons and funnels it into the ureter.

Major Calyx (plural: calyces)   A major calyx is a large, cup-shaped extension of the renal pelvis. There are 2 – 3 major calyces in each renal pelvis.

Minor Calyx   Each major calyx has 8 – 18 smaller cup-shaped extensions called minor calyces. Each minor calyx receives urine from the collecting ducts of one renal pyramid.

RIGHT KIDNEY
Coronal Section

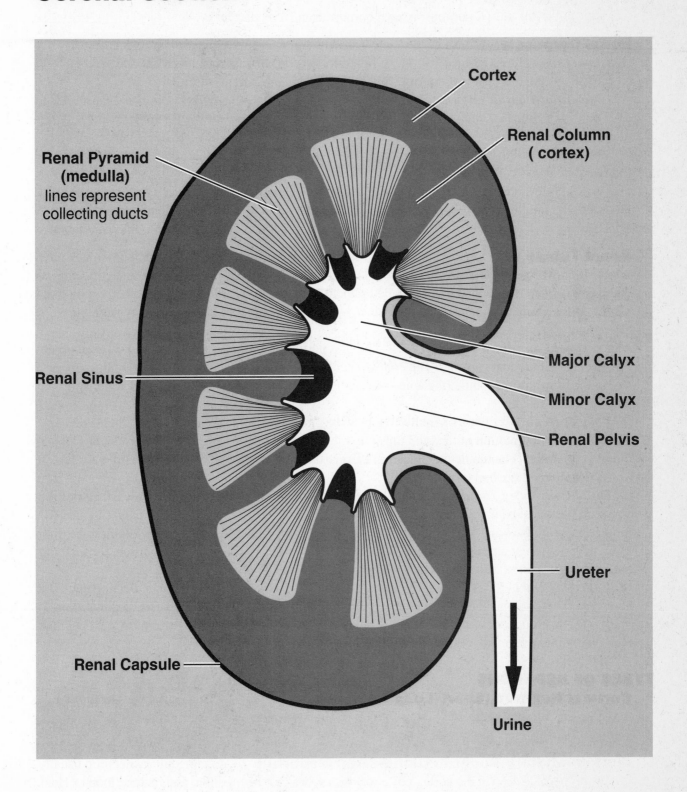

Cortex

Renal Column
(cortex)

Renal Pyramid
(medulla)
lines represent
collecting ducts

Major Calyx

Renal Sinus

Minor Calyx

Renal Pelvis

Ureter

Renal Capsule

Urine

PARTS OF A NEPHRON

A nephron consists of two portions: a renal corpuscle and a renal tubule.

Renal Corpuscle   A renal corpuscle consists of a glomerulus and a glomerular capsule.
(1) Glomerulus (plural: glomeruli)   The glomerulus is a tuft of capillary loops. Blood enters a glomerulus through an afferent arteriole and exits through an efferent arteriole.
(2) Glomerular Capsule (Bowman's Capsule)   The glomerular capsule (or Bowman's capsule) is a double-walled epithelial cup that surrounds the glomerulus. The *parietal layer* (outer wall) is separated from the *visceral layer* (inner wall) by the *capsular space* (Bowman's space). The epithelial cells of the visceral layer, called *podocytes*, are highly specialized for filtering the blood; they have footlike extensions called *pedicels*.

As blood flows through the glomerular capillaries, water and most kinds of solutes filter from blood plasma into the capsular space. Large plasma proteins and blood cells do not pass through. This process is called *filtration*. From the capsular space, filtered fluid passes into the renal tubule.

Renal Tubule   The renal tubule has four main sections. Fluid passes through them in this order: proximal convoluted tubule (PCT), loop of Henle, distal convoluted tubule (DCT), and collecting duct. *Convoluted* means the tubule is coiled rather than straight; *proximal* signifies the portion that is nearest to the glomerular capsule; and *distal* signifies the portion that is farthest away from the glomerular capsule.
(1) Proximal Convoluted Tubule (PCT)   The first portion of the renal tubule. The PCT is continuous with the glomerular capsule. The epithelial cells lining the PCT have microvilli on the surface facing the lumen of the tubule (the apical surface); this facilitates the reabsorption of water and nutrients.
(2) Loop of Henle   The loop of Henle connects the proximal and distal convoluted tubules of a nephron. The first portion of the loop dips into the medulla, where it is called the *descending limb* of the loop of Henle. The tubule then makes a hairpin turn and extends upward to the cortex as the *ascending limb* of the loop of Henle.
(3) Distal Convoluted Tubule (DCT)   When the ascending limb of the loop of Henle penetrates the cortex, it becomes the highly coiled distal convoluted tubule (DCT). As the DCT passes by the glomerulus, it makes contact with the blood vessels carrying blood to and from the glomerulus (the afferent and efferent arterioles). The cells in this portion of the DCT become modified, forming the *macula densa* (part of a structure called the *juxtaglomerular apparatus*).
(4) Collecting Duct   Several distal convoluted tubules empty urine into a single collecting duct. In each renal pyramid, many collecting ducts empty urine into about 30 larger ducts called *papillary ducts*. The papillary ducts widen gradually as they approach the tips of the pyramids (renal papillae); they empty into minor calyces of the renal pelvis.

TYPES OF NEPHRONS

Cortical Nephron (Short–Loop Nephron)   A cortical nephron usually has its glomerulus in the outer portion of the cortex; its short loop of Henle penetrates the outer region of the medulla. About 80% of the nephrons are of this type.

Juxtamedullary Nephron (Long–Loop Nephron)   A juxtamedullary nephron usually has its glomerulus deep in the cortex close to (*juxta* = beside) the medulla, and its long loop of Henle stretches through the medulla and almost reaches the renal papilla. These nephrons help regulate urine concentration. About 20% of the nephrons are of this type.

RENAL CORPUSCLE

The renal corpuscle has two components :
glomerulus (tuft of capillaries) and glomerular capsule (Bowman's capsule).

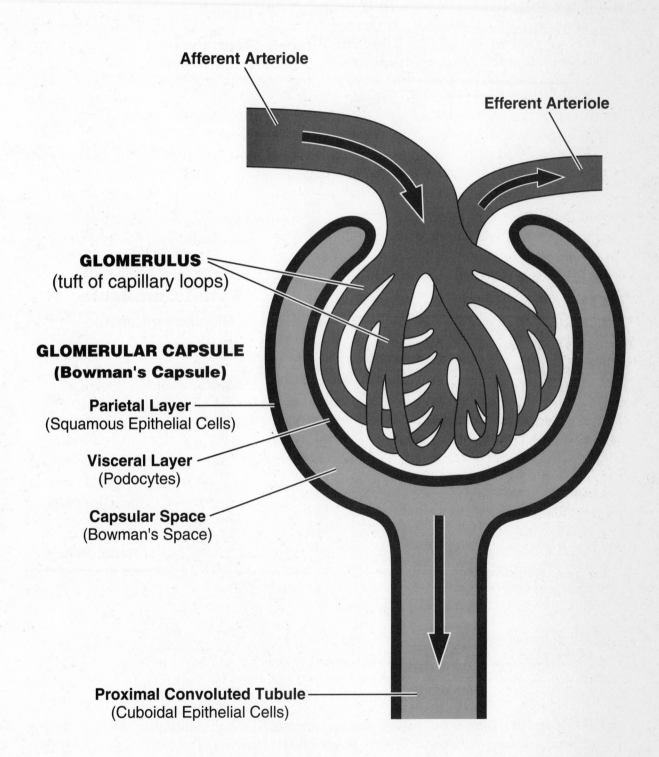

Afferent Arteriole

Efferent Arteriole

GLOMERULUS
(tuft of capillary loops)

GLOMERULAR CAPSULE
(Bowman's Capsule)

Parietal Layer
(Squamous Epithelial Cells)

Visceral Layer
(Podocytes)

Capsular Space
(Bowman's Space)

Proximal Convoluted Tubule
(Cuboidal Epithelial Cells)

CORTICAL NEPHRON

Location

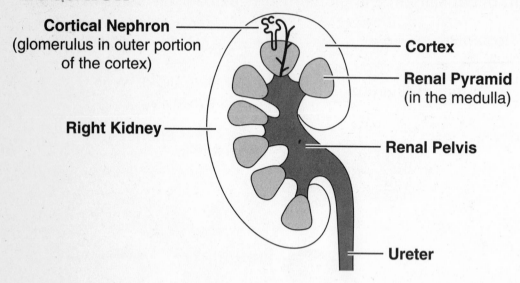

Cortical Nephron
(glomerulus in outer portion
of the cortex)

Right Kidney

Cortex

Renal Pyramid
(in the medulla)

Renal Pelvis

Ureter

Parts

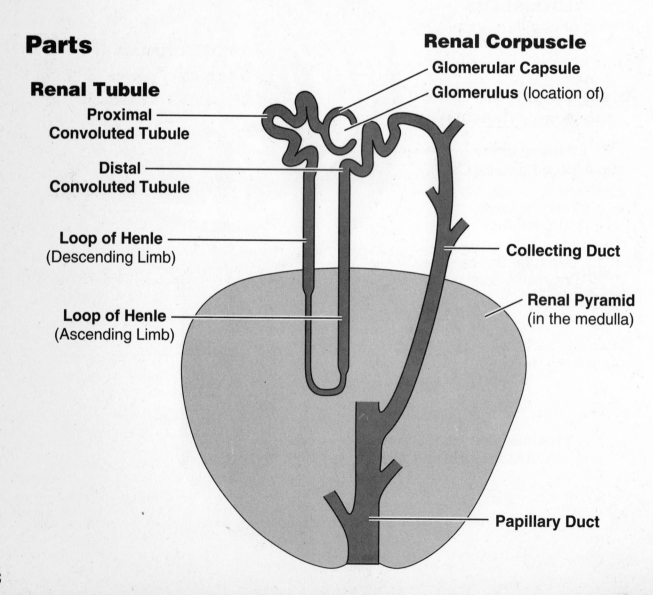

Renal Corpuscle

Glomerular Capsule

Glomerulus (location of)

Renal Tubule

Proximal
Convoluted Tubule

Distal
Convoluted Tubule

Loop of Henle
(Descending Limb)

Loop of Henle
(Ascending Limb)

Collecting Duct

Renal Pyramid
(in the medulla)

Papillary Duct

JUXTAMEDULLARY NEPHRON

Location

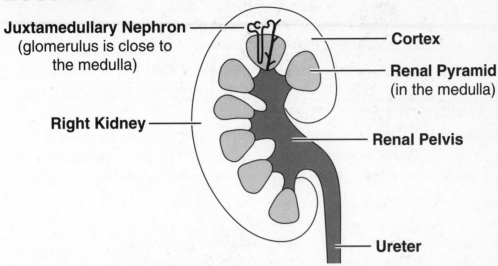

Juxtamedullary Nephron
(glomerulus is close to
the medulla)

Cortex

Renal Pyramid
(in the medulla)

Right Kidney

Renal Pelvis

Ureter

Parts

Renal Corpuscle

Renal Tubule

Glomerular Capsule

Glomerulus (location of)

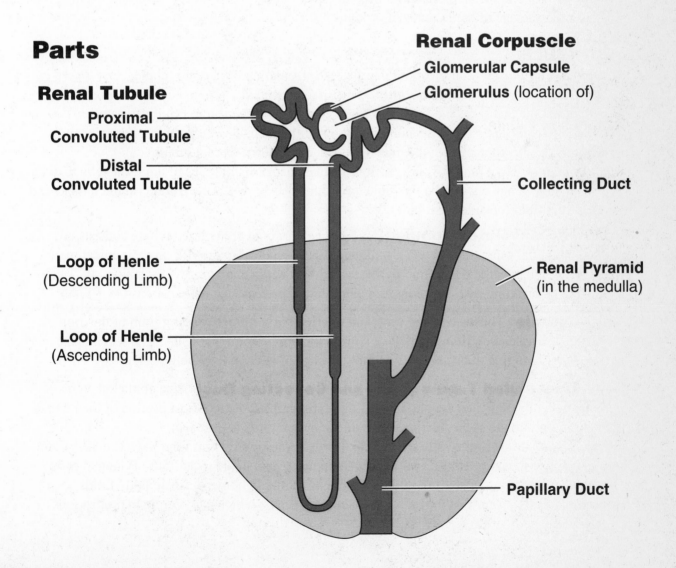

Proximal
Convoluted Tubule

Distal
Convoluted Tubule

Collecting Duct

Loop of Henle
(Descending Limb)

Renal Pyramid
(in the medulla)

Loop of Henle
(Ascending Limb)

Papillary Duct

STRUCTURES AND FUNCTIONS / Nephron Histology

ENDOTHELIAL–CAPSULAR MEMBRANE

The structure in the renal corpuscle that filters blood is called the endothelial-capsular membrane. Filtered substances pass through fenestrations (pores) in the glomerular endothelium, the basement membrane, and filtration slits formed by podocytes.

Endothelium   The endothelium is a layer of simple squamous epithelial cells that line the glomerular capillaries. This layer of cells has fenestrations (pores) averaging 50 to 100 nm in diameter, which restrict the passage of blood cells.

Basement Membrane   The basement membrane is a layer of extracellular material secreted by epithelial cells (endothelium and podocytes). It lies between the endothelium and the visceral layer of the glomerular capsule. It restricts the passage of large proteins.

Podocytes   Podocytes are specialized epithelial cells that form the visceral layer of the glomerular capsule.
Pedicels   Pedicels are footlike structures that extend out from the podocytes.
Filtration Slits   Filtration slits (slit pores) are spaces between the pedicels.
Slit Membrane   The slit membrane is a thin membrane that extends across a filtration slit, restricting the passage of medium-sized proteins.

RENAL TUBULE

Peritubular Capillaries   A network of capillaries surrounding each renal tubule.
Apical Membrane (Luminal Membrane)   The tip (apex) of an epithelial cell. The portion of the plasma membrane that faces the lumen and is in contact with the filtered fluid (filtrate).
Basolateral Membrane   The base and sides of an epithelial cell. The portion of the plasma membrane that is in contact with the interstitial fluid (outside the renal tubule).
Tight Junctions   Tight junctions are portions of the plasma membranes of adjacent cells that are in close contact. They restrict the movement of molecules between the filtrate (in the lumen) and the interstitial fluid (outside the tubule).

Proximal Convoluted Tubule (PCT)   The proximal convoluted tubule consists of cuboidal epithelial cells; they have a prominent brush border of microvilli on their apical membrane (facing the lumen). These microvilli increase the surface area for reabsorption. PCT cells are capable of secreting hydrogen ions and ammonium ions into the filtrate.

Loop of Henle   The descending limb and the first part of the ascending limb of the loop of Henle (the thin ascending limb) consist of simple squamous epithelial cells. The second part of the ascending limb (the thick ascending limb) consists of cuboidal epithelial cells.

Distal Convoluted Tubule (DCT) and Collecting Duct   The epithelial cells of the DCT and collecting duct are cuboidal. Beginning in the *late DCT* (last portion of the tubule) and continuing into the *collecting duct*, two different cell types are present.
Principal Cells   Most of the cells are principal cells. Antidiuretic hormone (ADH) makes them more permeable to water; aldosterone makes them more permeable to sodium. Principal cells are capable of secreting potassium into the filtrate to maintain homeostasis in body fluids.
Intercalated Cells   A few of the cells are intercalated cells, which can secrete hydrogen ions (H^+) to rid the body of excess acids.

ENDOTHELIAL – CAPSULAR MEMBRANE

Renal Corpuscle

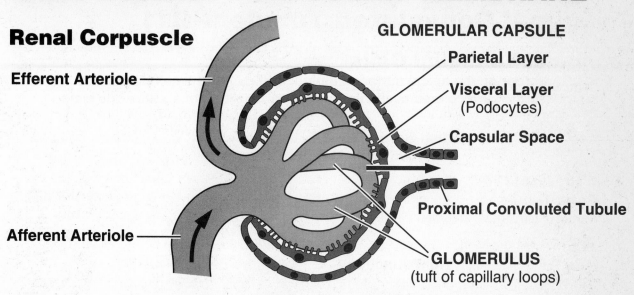

Efferent Arteriole

GLOMERULAR CAPSULE
Parietal Layer
Visceral Layer
(Podocytes)
Capsular Space

Proximal Convoluted Tubule

Afferent Arteriole

GLOMERULUS
(tuft of capillary loops)

Podocytes

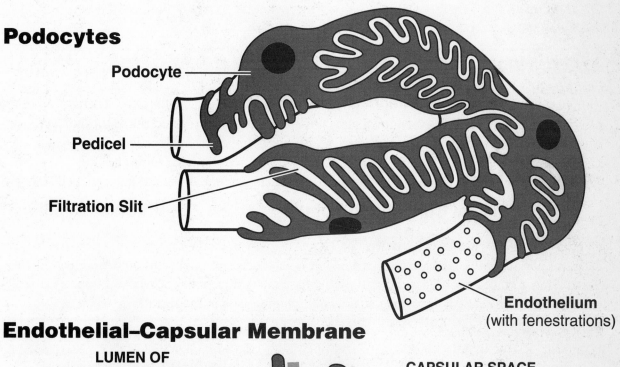

Podocyte

Pedicel

Filtration Slit

Endothelium
(with fenestrations)

Endothelial–Capsular Membrane

LUMEN OF
GLOMERULAR CAPILLARY

CAPSULAR SPACE

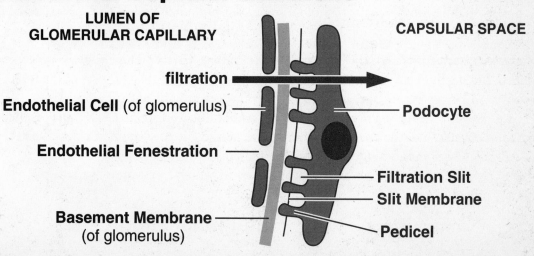

filtration

Endothelial Cell (of glomerulus)

Podocyte

Endothelial Fenestration

Filtration Slit
Slit Membrane

Basement Membrane
(of glomerulus)

Pedicel

11

RENAL TUBULE HISTOLOGY :
Proximal Convoluted Tubule (PCT)

Cuboidal Epithelial Cells

The brush border on the apical surface (luminal surface) of the cells lining the PCT increase the surface area available for the reabsorption of solutes and water.

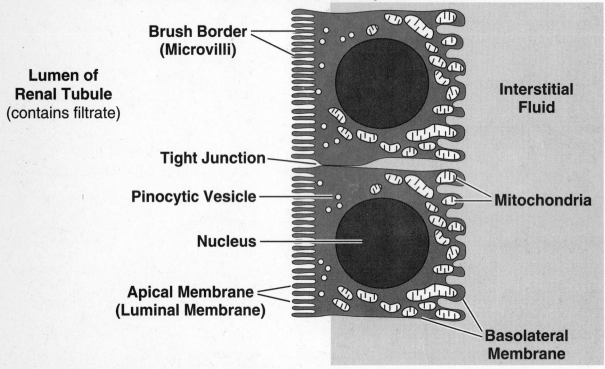

Brush Border (Microvilli)

Lumen of Renal Tubule (contains filtrate)

Interstitial Fluid

Tight Junction

Pinocytic Vesicle

Mitochondria

Nucleus

Apical Membrane (Luminal Membrane)

Basolateral Membrane

Cross Section of the PCT

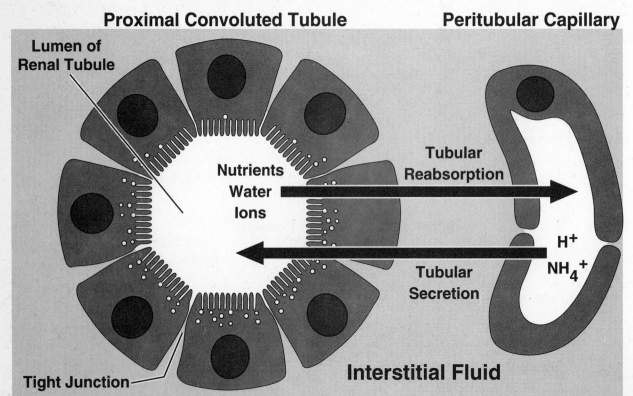

Proximal Convoluted Tubule

Peritubular Capillary

Lumen of Renal Tubule

Nutrients
Water
Ions

Tubular Reabsorption

H^+
NH_4^+

Tubular Secretion

Tight Junction

Interstitial Fluid

RENAL TUBULE HISTOLOGY :
Distal Convoluted Tubule (DCT) and Collecting Duct
Cuboidal Epithelial Cells

Most of the cells lining the DCT and collecting ducts are called **Principal Cells**. Antidiuretic hormone (ADH) makes their apical membranes permeable to water. Principal cells are capable of secreting potassium ions.

Some of the cells lining the DCT and collecting ducts are called **Intercalated Cells**. They are capable of secreting hydrogen ions.

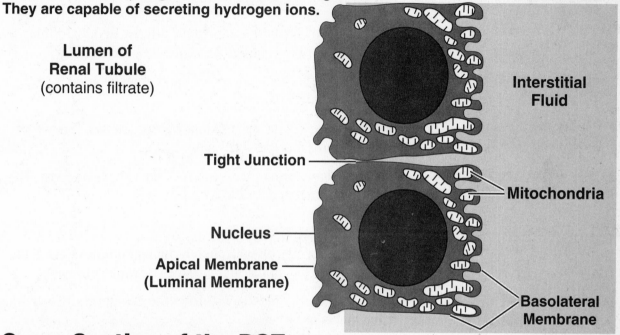

Lumen of
Renal Tubule
(contains filtrate)

Interstitial
Fluid

Tight Junction

Mitochondria

Nucleus

Apical Membrane
(Luminal Membrane)

Basolateral
Membrane

Cross Section of the DCT

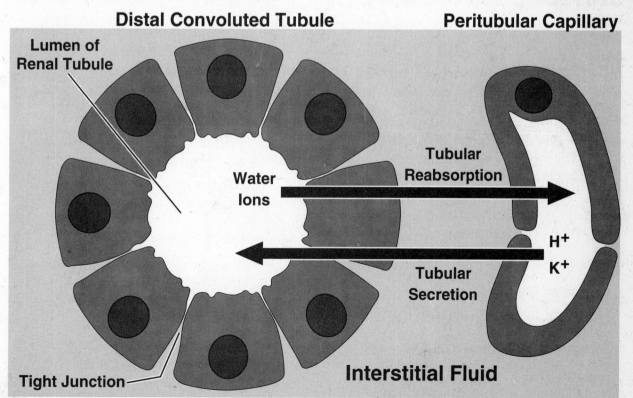

Distal Convoluted Tubule

Peritubular Capillary

Lumen of
Renal Tubule

Water
Ions

Tubular
Reabsorption

H^+
K^+

Tubular
Secretion

Tight Junction

Interstitial Fluid

STRUCTURES AND FUNCTIONS / Kidney Blood Supply

Approximately 25% of the cardiac output (about 1200 ml of blood per minute) passes through the kidneys. About 20% of the fluid portion of this blood (plasma) is filtered; it enters the renal tubules and is converted into urine.

ARTERIES

Renal Arteries The right and left renal arteries carry blood from the abdominal aorta to the right and left kidneys.

Segmental Arteries In each kidney, the branches of the renal arteries divide, forming five segmental arteries. Each segmental artery supplies a particular segment of a kidney.

Interlobar Arteries The interlobar arteries are branches of the segmental arteries. They pass through the renal columns (between the renal pyramids).

Arcuate Arteries The arcuate arteries are branches of the interlobar arteries. They form arches between the bases of the renal pyramids and the outer cortex.

Interlobular Arteries The interlobular arteries are divisions of the arcuate arteries. They extend into the outer cortex and divide into afferent arterioles.

ARTERIOLES

Afferent Arterioles Afferent arterioles carry blood from interlobular arteries toward the glomerulus (a ball of capillaries located inside the glomerular capsule (Bowman's capsule).

Efferent Arterioles Efferent arterioles carry blood away from the glomerulus. They drain the glomerular capillaries of the blood that is not filtered.

CAPILLARIES

Glomerulus (Glomerular Capillaries) The glomerulus is a tuft of capillary loops located inside the glomerular capsule. Blood filters from the glomerulus into the capsular space.

Peritubular Capillaries Peritubular capillaries are a network of capillaries that surround the PCT and DCT. They drain blood from the efferent arterioles. Nutrients, ions, and water are reabsorbed from the PCT and DCT into the peritubular capillaries.

Vasa Recta The vasa recta are long, straight, loop-shaped capillaries that dip down alongside the loop of Henle in juxtamedullary (long-loop) nephrons. The vasa recta are important in the formation of concentrated urine.

VEINS

Peritubular Venules Drain the peritubular capillaries and the vasa recta.

Interlobular Veins Drain the peritubular venules.

Arcuate Veins Drain the interlobular veins.

Interlobar Veins Drain the Arcuate veins. Run between the renal pyramids.

Segmental Veins Drain the interlobar veins.

Renal Veins Drain the segmental veins and empty into the inferior vena cava.

BLOOD SUPPLY TO KIDNEY

Only the arteries are shown in this illustration. The veins run parallel to the arteries and have the same names.

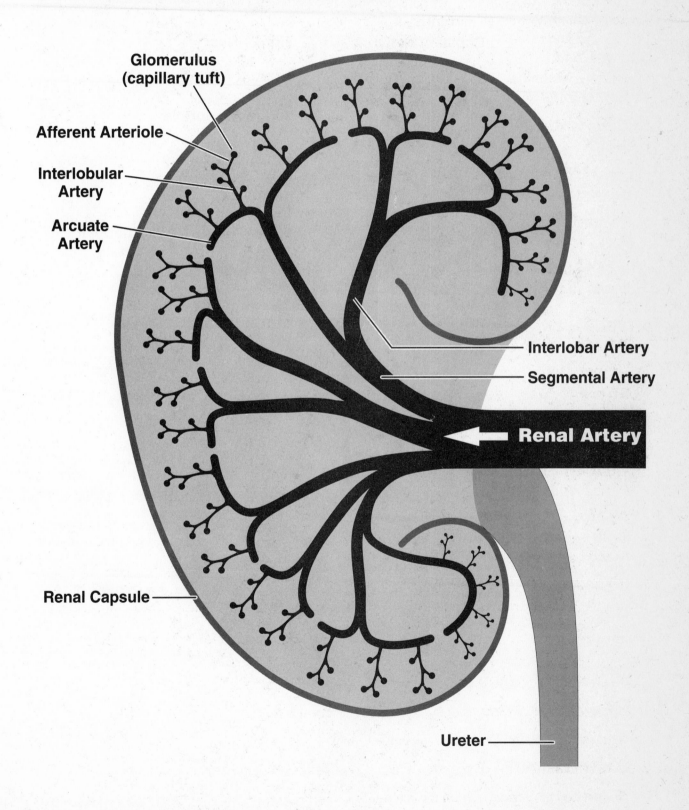

Glomerulus (capillary tuft)

Afferent Arteriole

Interlobular Artery

Arcuate Artery

Interlobar Artery

Segmental Artery

Renal Artery

Renal Capsule

Ureter

CORTICAL NEPHRON
Blood Supply

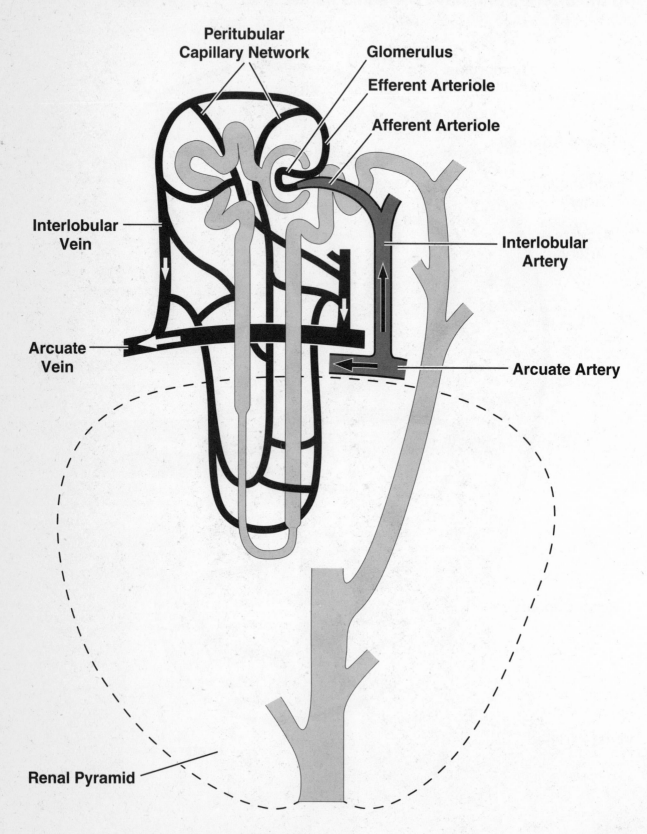

Peritubular
Capillary Network

Glomerulus

Efferent Arteriole

Afferent Arteriole

Interlobular
Vein

Interlobular
Artery

Arcuate
Vein

Arcuate Artery

Renal Pyramid

JUXTAMEDULLARY NEPHRON
Blood Supply

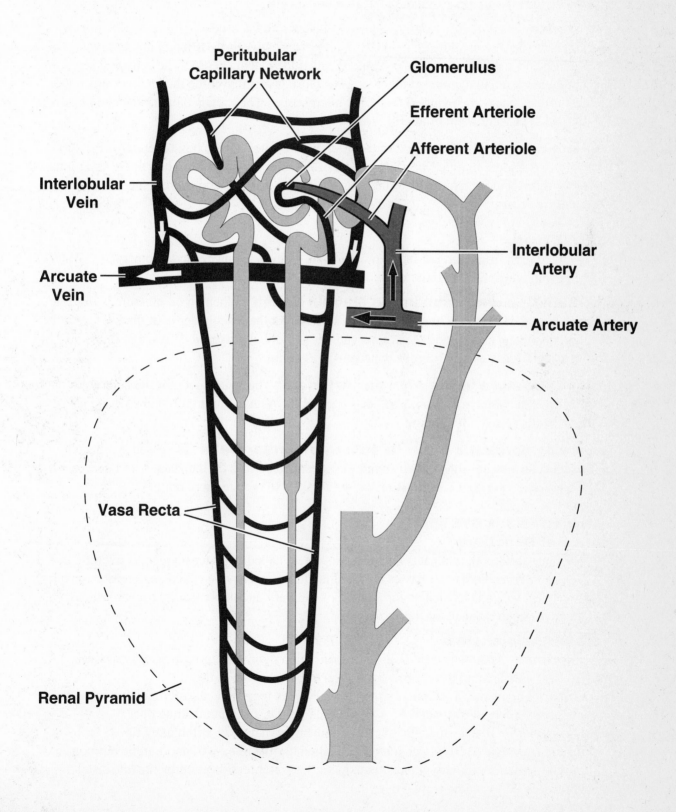

Peritubular Capillary Network

Glomerulus

Efferent Arteriole

Afferent Arteriole

Interlobular Vein

Interlobular Artery

Arcuate Vein

Arcuate Artery

Vasa Recta

Renal Pyramid

RENAL PHYSIOLOGY / Juxtaglomerular Apparatus

STRUCTURES

The juxtaglomerular apparatus (JGA) is a structure located next to (*juxta* = beside) the glomerulus of each nephron. The JGA helps regulate blood pressure and the rate of blood filtration by the kidneys. It has two parts, the macula densa and the juxtaglomerular cells.

Macula Densa (*macula* = spot; *densa* = dense) Just before the ascending limb of the loop of Henle becomes the distal convoluted tubule (DCT), it passes between the afferent and efferent arterioles. This short segment of the renal tubule is called the macula densa. The cells in this region of the renal tubule are tall and crowded together. The close proximity of the nuclei gives this region a dense (dark) appearance when viewed by a light microscope. These cells monitor the rate of flow and the salt (NaCl) concentration of the filtrate.

Juxtaglomerular Cells A portion of the afferent arteriole. The juxtaglomerular cells (JG cells) are modified smooth muscle fibers in the wall of the afferent arteriole. Their nuclei are round and their cytoplasm includes renin-containing granules. In response to the appropriate stimuli, they secrete the enzyme renin.

RENIN SECRETION

Renin is involved in the regulation of blood pressure and sodium balance. Juxtaglomerular cells (JG cells) secrete renin in response to three kinds of stimuli.

Low Sodium Concentration in the Macula Densa When blood pressure is low, the rate of filtration in the kidneys is low. Fluid flows slowly past the macula densa of the DCT, and the concentration of sodium and chloride ions (Na^+ and Cl^-) is low. Decreased delivery of fluid and NaCl to the macula densa causes JG cells to secrete more renin.

Low Blood Pressure in the Afferent Arteriole The renin-secreting JG cells are pressure sensitive; they function as intrarenal baroreceptors. As renal arterial blood pressure decreases, the JG cells secrete more renin.

Increased Sympathetic Input to Juxtaglomerular Cells Increased sympathetic input to the JG cells may be stimulated by exercise, stress, blood loss (hemorrhage), or a decrease in the blood pressure. Sympathetic stimulation causes JG cells to secrete more renin.

RENIN–ANGIOTENSIN SYSTEM
Sequence of Reactions

Once released into the blood, renin acts on a plasma protein called angiotensinogen, converting it into angiotensin I. As angiotensin I passes through the lungs, an enzyme called angiotensin converting enzyme (ACE), which is located on the surface of capillary endothelial cells, converts angiotensin I into angiotensin II (an active hormone).

Actions of Angiotensin II

(1) Vasoconstriction Angiotensin II causes the constriction of efferent arterioles; this elevates glomerular blood pressure and increases the filtration of blood in the kidneys.

(2) Aldosterone Angiotensin II stimulates the adrenal cortex to secrete aldosterone; this enhances reabsorption of sodium by the *late* distal convoluted tubule (DCT) and collecting duct.

(3) Thirst Angiotensin II acts on the thirst center in the hypothalamus, stimulating thirst.

(4) Antidiuretic Hormone (ADH) Angiotensin II stimulates the release of antidiuretic hormone (ADH) from the posterior pituitary gland, which increases water reabsorption by the *late* distal convoluted tubule (DCT) and collecting duct.

JUXTAGLOMERULAR APPARATUS

Juxtaglomerular Apparatus :
The juxtaglomerular apparatus is located next to (juxta) the glomerulus.
It has two parts, the juxtaglomeruluar cells and the macula densa.

Juxtaglomerular Cells :
Modified smooth muscle cells of the afferent arteriole.
They secrete the enzyme renin.

Macula Densa :
Specialized cells of the distal convoluted tubule.
They are sensitive to sodium concentrations in the filtrate.

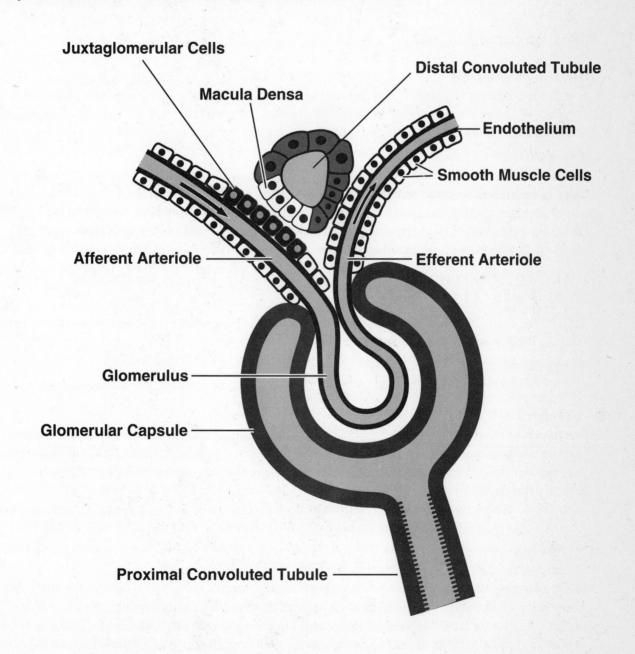

STRUCTURES AND FUNCTIONS / Ureters, Urinary Bladder, and Urethra

URETERS

There are two ureters—one for each kidney. Each ureter is an extension of the renal pelvis and stretches about 12 inches to the urinary bladder. The widest portion of a ureter has a diameter of about 0.5 inch. The ureters are *retroperitoneal* structures (located behind the peritoneum).

Structure

Tissue Layers Three coats of tissue form the walls of the ureters. They are, from the inside out, the mucosa, the muscularis, and the serosa. The *mucosa* consists of transitional epithelium. Throughout most of the length of the ureters, the *muscularis* is composed of inner longitudinal and outer circular layers of smooth muscle. The external coat, the *serosa*, is a layer of fibrous connective tissue.

Function

Urine Transport Peristalsis moves urine through the ureters to the bladder.

URINARY BLADDER

The urinary bladder is a hollow muscular organ located in the pelvic cavity posterior to the pubic symphysis. It is a retroperitoneal structure. In the male, it is directly anterior to the rectum; in the female, it is anterior to the vagina and inferior to the uterus. Capacity: 700 to 800 ml.

Structures

Tissue Layers Three coats of tissue form the wall of the urinary bladder. They are, from deep to superficial: the mucosa, the detrusor muscle, and the serosa. The *mucosa* consists of transitional epithelium, which allows it to stretch, and an underlying layer of connective tissue (the lamina propria). *Rugae* (folds in the mucosa) are also present. Mucus protects the cells from urine. The *detrusor muscle* consists of three layers of smooth muscle. Fibers of the detrusor muscle surround the opening to the urethra, forming the *internal urethral sphincter*. The outer coat, the serosa, is a layer of fibrous connective tissue. The superior surface of the bladder is covered by the *peritoneum*.
Trigone The trigone is a small triangular area in the floor of the bladder. The two posterior corners contain the *ureteral openings* (openings to the two ureters); the anterior corner contains the *internal urethral orifice* (opening to the urethra).

Functions

Storage and Micturition The bladder stores urine and contracts during micturition (urination).

URETHRA

The urethra is a small tube leading from the floor of the urinary bladder to the exterior of the body. It is about 8 inches long in the male and 1.5 inches long in the female. A modification of the urogenital diaphragm (skeletal muscle) forms the *external urethral sphincter* (under voluntary control).

Male Urethra

Structures The wall of the urethra consists of two coats: an inner *mucous membrane* and an outer *submucous tissue*. The opening of the urethra to the exterior is called the *external urethral orifice*.
Functions The male urethra serves as a passageway for eliminating urine and a duct through which semen is discharged from the body during sexual intercourse.

Female Urethra

Structures The wall of the female urethra consists of three coats: an inner coat, the *mucosa*; a middle coat, a thin layer of spongy tissue containing a plexus of veins; and an outer coat, the *serosa*, which is continuous with the serosa of the urinary bladder. The opening of the urethra to the exterior is called the *external urethral orifice*; it is located between the clitoris and the vaginal opening.
Function The female urethra serves as a passageway for eliminating urine from the body.

URINARY BLADDER AND URETHRA
Coronal Section (Female)

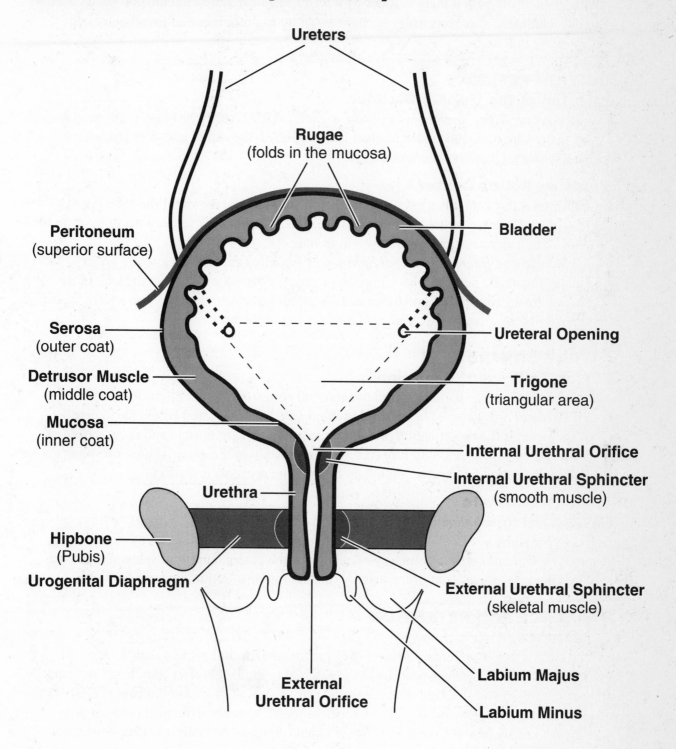

Ureters

Rugae
(folds in the mucosa)

Bladder

Peritoneum
(superior surface)

Serosa
(outer coat)

Ureteral Opening

Detrusor Muscle
(middle coat)

Trigone
(triangular area)

Mucosa
(inner coat)

Internal Urethral Orifice

Internal Urethral Sphincter
(smooth muscle)

Urethra

Hipbone
(Pubis)

Urogenital Diaphragm

External Urethral Sphincter
(skeletal muscle)

Labium Majus

External
Urethral Orifice

Labium Minus

Urine is expelled from the urinary bladder by a reflex response called micturition (also called urination or voiding). This response is brought about by a combination of involuntary and voluntary nerve imlpulses.

MICTURITION REFLEX
Distension of the Urinary Bladder
Stretch Receptors   When the amount of urine in the bladder exceeds 200 to 400 ml, stretch receptors in the wall of the distended bladder are stimulated; they send impulses via sensory neurons to the sacral region of the spinal cord.

Micturition Reflex Center
The micturition reflex center is a network of neurons in the sacral region of the spinal cord.
Brain (Cerebral Cortex)   Impulses are sent to the cerebral cortex via sensory nerve tracts in the spinal cord. They initiate a conscious desire to urinate.
Detrusor Muscle and Internal Urethral Sphincter   Impulses are sent back to the urinary bladder via parasympathetic nerves. These impulses cause the detrusor muscle in the wall of the bladder to contract rhythmically and the internal urethral sphincter to relax. The internal urethral sphincter is a ring of smooth muscle around the opening of the urethra.

VOLUNTARY CONTROL
Decision To Prevent Urination
Brain (Cerebral Cortex)   Impulses from the cerebral cortex inhibit the micturition reflex.
External Urethral Sphincter   The external urethral sphincter is located below the internal urethral sphincter; it is a modification of the urogenital diaphragm muscle and is composed of skeletal muscle, so it is under voluntary control. Contraction of the external urethral sphincter is controlled by the pudendal nerves. Voluntary contraction prevents urination.

Decision To Urinate
Brain (Pons and Hypothalamus)   The micturition reflex is facilitated by impulses from the pons and hypothalamus.
External Urethral Sphincter   Voluntary relaxation of the external urethral sphincter (skeletal muscle) allows urine to pass out of the urinary bladder into the urethra, and out of the body.

INCONTINENCE AND RETENTION
Incontinence
Incontinence is a lack of voluntary control over micturition. In infants less than 2 years old, incontinence is normal, because neurons to the external urethral sphincter muscle are not completely developed. In adults, incontinence may occur as a result of unconsciousness, injury to the spinal nerves controlling the urinary bladder, irritation due to abnormal constituents in urine, disease of the urinary bladder, damage to the external sphincter, or inability of the detrusor muscle to relax (caused by tension due to emotional stress).

Retention
Retention is a failure to completely or normally void urine. It may be caused by an obstruction in the urethra or neck of the urinary bladder, nervous contraction of the urethra, or lack of sensation to urinate.

MICTURITION

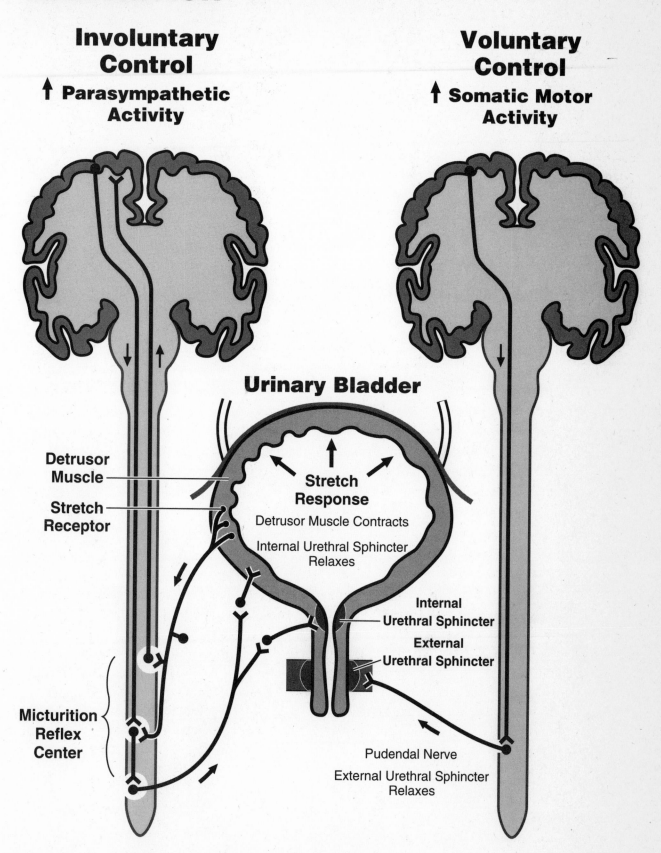

Involuntary Control
↑ Parasympathetic Activity

Voluntary Control
↑ Somatic Motor Activity

Urinary Bladder

Detrusor Muscle

Stretch Receptor

Stretch Response

Detrusor Muscle Contracts

Internal Urethral Sphincter Relaxes

Internal Urethral Sphincter

External Urethral Sphincter

Micturition Reflex Center

Pudendal Nerve

External Urethral Sphincter Relaxes

2 Urine Formation

URINE FORMATION / Overview

RENAL PROCESSES

Urine formation occurs in the nephrons and involves three basic processes: (1) glomerular filtration, (2) tubular reabsorption, and (3) tubular secretion.

Glomerular Filtration

The first step in the formation of urine is glomerular filtration. Each day about 180 liters of protein-free blood plasma pass from the glomeruli of both kidneys into the renal tubules. Once in the renal tubules, the blood plasma is called *glomerular filtrate*. The filtration process is driven by the hydrostatic pressure (blood pressure) in the glomerular capillaries. It is opposed by two forces: the hydrostatic pressure in the glomerular capsule and the osmotic force that is due to the presence of plasma proteins in the glomerular capillaries.

Tubular Reabsorption

As filtrate passes through the renal tubules, substances that are useful to the body are returned to the capillaries surrounding the tubules (peritubular capillaries) by a process called tubular reabsorption. About 99% of the water, sodium, and glucose is reabsorbed; only about 44% of the urea (toxic nitrogenous waste) is reabsorbed.

Tubular Secretion

The movement of substances from the peritubular capillaries into the renal tubules is called tubular secretion. Certain ions (hydrogen ions, potassium ions, and ammonium ions), nitrogenous wastes (urea, creatinine, and uric acid), and certain drugs (such as penicillin) may be secreted into the filtrate from the blood in the peritubular capillaries.

RENAL FUNCTIONS

Nephrons carry out three important functions: (1) control of blood concentration and volume; (2) control of blood pH; and (3) removal of toxic wastes from the blood.

Control of Blood Concentration and Volume

Nephrons control blood concentration and volume by removing selected amounts of water and solutes (especially ions) from the blood.

Control of Blood pH

When the blood becomes too acidic, excess hydrogen ions are secreted into the filtrate and excreted in the urine; bicarbonate ions (weak bases) are reabsorbed.

Removal of Toxic Wastes

The breakdown (catabolism) of nitrogen-containing compounds in the cells produces toxic wastes, which are excreted in the urine. Urea is derived from the deamination of amino acids to form ammonia (the liver converts ammonia into urea); creatinine is derived from the breakdown of creatine phosphate (nitrogenous substance in muscle tissue); uric acid is derived from the breakdown of nucleic acids (RNA and DNA).

URINE

Water accounts for about 95% of the total volume of urine. The remaining 5% consists of organic and inorganic solutes. In the normal adult, the volume of urine eliminated per day is about 1 to 2 quarts (1 to 2 liters).

URINE FORMATION
Diagrammatic

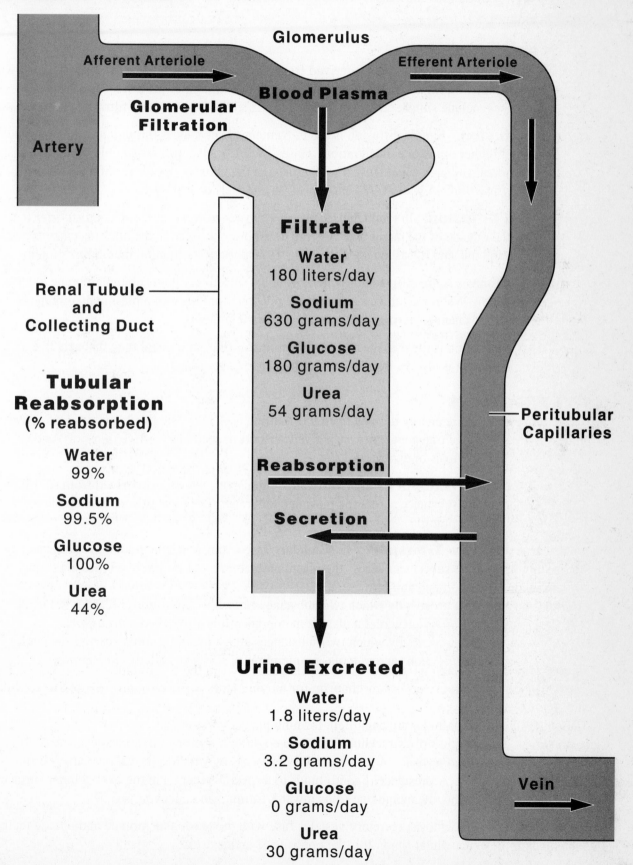

Glomerulus

Afferent Arteriole

Efferent Arteriole

Blood Plasma

Glomerular Filtration

Artery

Renal Tubule
and
Collecting Duct

Filtrate

Water
180 liters/day

Sodium
630 grams/day

Glucose
180 grams/day

Urea
54 grams/day

Tubular Reabsorption
(% reabsorbed)

Water
99%

Sodium
99.5%

Glucose
100%

Urea
44%

Reabsorption

Secretion

Peritubular Capillaries

Urine Excreted

Water
1.8 liters/day

Sodium
3.2 grams/day

Glucose
0 grams/day

Urea
30 grams/day

Vein

URINE FORMATION / Membrane Transport

The mechanisms that move substances across cell membranes may be passive (do not require ATP) or active (require ATP).

PASSIVE PROCESSES

Passive processes do not require energy derived from the splitting of ATP. Substances move down a concentration gradient from an area of higher to lower concentration or pressure. The basic types of passive processes include simple diffusion, facilitated diffusion, osmosis, and filtration.

Simple Diffusion   Simple diffusion is the movement of substances through a cell membrane from an area of higher to lower concentration. Gases, steroids, glycerol, fat-soluble vitamins, small alcohols, ammonia, and urea can diffuse directly through the phospholipid layer of a plasma membrane. Ions diffuse through water-filled channels (ion channels or pores).

Facilitated Diffusion   In facilitated diffusion a substance combines with a *transporter* (carrier molecule) on the outside of the membrane. As the transporter changes shape, the substance is carried through the membrane and released inside the cell. Transporters are integral membrane proteins.

Osmosis   Osmosis is the diffusion of water through a selectively permeable membrane (such as a plasma membrane). Water may diffuse through the phospholipid layer of a plasma membrane or through water-filled channels formed by integral membrane proteins.

Filtration   Filtration is the passage of a liquid through a filter or a membrane that acts like a filter. Such movement is always from an area of higher to lower pressure.

ACTIVE PROCESSES

Active processes require energy derived from the splitting of ATP. The two basic types of active processes are: (1) active transport (primary active transport or secondary active transport) and (2) bulk transport (endocytosis or exocytosis).

Primary Active Transport   In primary active transport, the energy derived from splitting ATP *directly* moves a substance across the plasma membrane. The most prevalent example is the sodium pump (Na^+/K^+ pump).

Secondary Active Transport   In secondary active transport, ion gradients established by the sodium pump drive substances across the plasma membrane. There are two types of secondary active transport: symport and antiport.
Symport   Symport is a process by which two substances attach to a transporter (carrier molecule) and move in the *same direction* across a plasma membrane. It is also called *cotransport*.
Antiport   Antiport is a process by which two substances attach to a transporter (carrier molecule) and move in *opposite directions* across a plasma membrane. It is also called *countertransport*.

Endocytosis   Endocytosis is a mechanism for moving large particles or droplets of extracellular fluid into cells.
Phagocytosis   Large particles are englulfed, forming phagocytic vesicles.
Pinocytosis   Tiny droplets of extracellular fluid are englulfed, forming pinocytic vesicles.
Receptor-mediated Endocytosis   A highly selective process by which cells can take up specific molecules or particles. A substance (ligand) binds to a specific receptor at the extracellular surface of the plasma membrane; the membrane folds inward, forming an endocytic vesicle.

Exocytosis   In exocytosis, secretory vesicles fuse with the plasma membrane and release their contents into the extracellular fluid. It is the opposite of endocytosis.

SODIUM PUMP (Na⁺ / K⁺ ATP–ase)

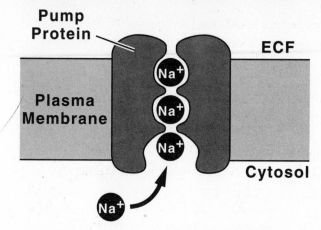

Sodium in the cytosol
binds to the pump protein.

Sodium concentration is low
in the cytosol relative to the ECF.

Potassium concentration is high
in the cytosol relative to the ECF.

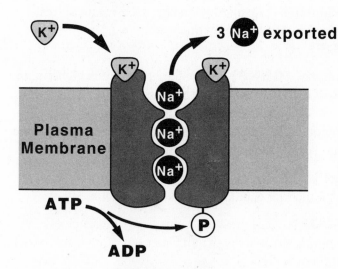

Na^+ binding triggers
the breakdown of ATP into ADP
and the attachment of a
high-energy phosphate group
to the pump protein.

This changes the shape of the
pump protein so that the sodium ions
are pushed through the membrane
and exported into the ECF.

Now the shape of the pump favors
binding of K^+ in the ECF.

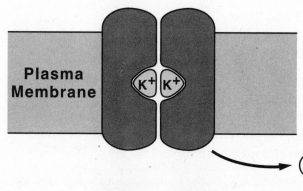

K^+ binding triggers
the release of phosphate, again causing
the shape of the pump protein to change.

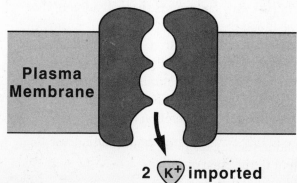

K^+ is pushed through the membrane
into the cytosol, as the pump
returns to its original shape.

The cycle repeats itself.

URINE FORMATION / Glomerular Filtration

Glomerular Filtration   Glomerular filtration, which occurs in the renal corpuscles of the kidneys, is the first step in the production of urine. Blood pressure forces water and solutes from glomerular capillaries, through the endothelial-capsular membrane, which acts as a filter, into the capsular space.
Filter   The endothelial-capsular membrane has three layers: the wall of the capillaries (glomerular endothelium), a basement membrane, and the visceral wall of the glomerular capsule.
Filtrate   The fluid that has been filtered is called the filtrate (also called the nephric filtrate or tubular fluid). Filtrate contains all the materials present in blood plasma except the plasma proteins, which are too large to pass through the endothelial-capsular membrane.
Filtration Fraction   The percentage of plasma that is filtered is called the filtration fraction.

NET FILTRATION PRESSURE (NFP)

The net pressure that promotes glomerular filtration is called the net filtration pressure (NFP). It is calculated by subtracting the forces that oppose filtration (capsular hydrostatic pressure and blood colloid osmotic pressure) from the glomerular blood hydrostatic pressure.

$$NFP = GBHP - (CHP + BCOP)$$

Glomerular Blood Hydrostatic Pressure (GBHP)   The blood pressure is higher in the glomerular capillaries than in capillaries elsewhere in the body. This is because the efferent arteriole is smaller in diameter than the afferent arteriole, so blood tends to back up in the glomerular capillaries due to the high resistance to the outflow of blood. Also, the arterioles leading to the glomeruli are short and offer little resistance to bloodflow. The GBHP is about 60 mm Hg.

Capsular Hydrostatic Pressure (CHP)   The hydrostatic pressure of the filtrate in the capsular space tends to push fluid back into the glomerular capillaries. It is about 15 mm Hg.

Blood Colloid Osmotic Pressure (BCOP)   This pressure is due to the presence of proteins in the blood plasma of the glomerular capillaries. It tends to pull water out of the filtrate back into the blood. The BCOP averages about 27 mm Hg.

GLOMERULAR FILTRATION RATE (GFR)

The amount of filtrate that forms in all the renal corpuscles of both kidneys every minute is called the glomerular filtration rate (GFR). In the normal adult the GFR is about 125 ml/min. Three mechanisms regulate the GFR: autoregulation, hormonal regulation, and neural regulation.

Renal Autoregulation   When the arterial blood pressure is low, a decreased amount of fluid and salt (NaCl) flows past the juxtaglomerular apparatus. This inhibits the release of vasoconstrictor substance from the juxtaglomerular cells. As a result, the afferent arterioles dilate, allowing more blood to flow into the glomerular capillaries, which increases the GBHP and the GFR.

Hormonal Regulation   When arterial blood pressure is low, the juxtaglomerular cells release the enzyme *renin*, which triggers the renin-angiotensin pathway, and causes the activation of the hormone *angiotensin II*. Angiotensin II helps raise the blood pressure and GFR by (1) causing the constriction of efferent arterioles; (2) stimulating the secretion of aldosterone, which enhances the reabsorption of sodium and therefore water by the principal cells of the collecting ducts; (3) stimulating thirst; and (4) stimulating the release of antidiuretic hormone, which stimulates the reabsorption of water from the collecting ducts. A second hormone that influences the GFR is atrial natriuretic peptide (ANP); it lowers blood pressure and GFR by promoting the excretion of water.

Neural Regulation   Strong sympathetic stimulation (during exercise, fight-or-flight response, or hemorrhage) lowers the GFR by causing constriction of the afferent arterioles.

NET FILTRATION PRESSURE

NFP = GBHP − (CHP + BCOP)

NFP = Net Filtration Pressure = 18 mm Hg

GBHP = Glomerular Blood Hydrostatic Pressure = 60 mm Hg

CHP = Capsular Hydrostatic Pressure = 15 mm Hg

BCOP = Blood Colloid Osmotic Pressure = 27 mm Hg

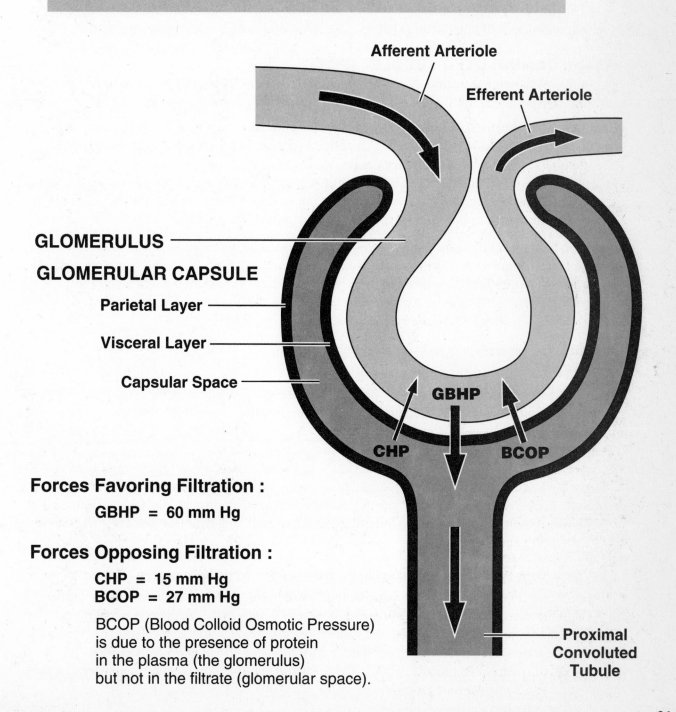

Afferent Arteriole

Efferent Arteriole

GLOMERULUS

GLOMERULAR CAPSULE

Parietal Layer

Visceral Layer

Capsular Space

GBHP

CHP

BCOP

Proximal Convoluted Tubule

Forces Favoring Filtration :

GBHP = 60 mm Hg

Forces Opposing Filtration :

CHP = 15 mm Hg
BCOP = 27 mm Hg

BCOP (Blood Colloid Osmotic Pressure)
is due to the presence of protein
in the plasma (the glomerulus)
but not in the filtrate (glomerular space).

URINE FORMATION / Tubular Reabsorption

Tubular Reabsorption   Tubular reabsorption is the movement of solutes and water from the filtrate (tubular fluid) back into the blood of the peritubular capillaries. Reabsorption is generally very high for nutrients, ions, and water; it is lower for waste products. About 99% of the filtrate is reabsorbed.
Mechanisms   Reabsorption occurs by passive processes (simple diffusion, facilitated diffusion, and osmosis) and active processes (primary active transport, secondary active transport, and pinocytosis).
Transport Maximum (T_m)   The transport maximum is the maximum amount of a substance that can be reabsorbed by renal tubules per minute. It is measured in mg/min. Each transport mechanism has an upper limit on how fast it can work. When the plasma concentration of a substance is abnormally high, there is not sufficient time for complete reabsorption; these substances appear in the urine.
Renal Threshold   The renal threshold is the plasma concentration (measured in mg/ml) at which a substance begins to spill into the urine because the transport maximum has been surpassed.

PROXIMAL CONVOLUTED TUBULE   (PCT)

Most of the reabsorption of nutrients and water takes place in the PCT; the brush border (microvilli) of the tubule cells lining the PCT greatly increases the surface area for reabsorption.

Nutrients   Normally 100% of the filtered glucose, amino acids, lactic acid, and other useful substances are reabsorbed from the PCT. All of these substances are transported into the tubule by Na^+ symporters, which work by secondary active transport. These substances leave the cells by facilitated diffusion through the basolateral membrane and then diffuse into peritubular capillaries. Small proteins and peptides are transported into the tubule cells by pinocytosis, and then are broken down into amino acids that are used by the cells or transported into the blood.

Ions   Sodium ions diffuse from the filtrate through leakage channels in the brush border (apical membrane) into tubule cells. At the same time, sodium pumps in the basolateral membrane actively transport sodium ions into the interstitial fluid. Sodium ions diffuse from the interstitial fluid into the peritubular capillaries. Concentration gradients generated by the osmosis of water promote the reabsorption of ions (potassium, chloride, and bicarbonate) by diffusion.

Water   The reabsorption of sodium ions generates an osmotic gradient, which causes the reabsorption of water by osmosis.

Wastes   Wastes such as urea are only partially reabsorbed. Only 44% of the urea in the filtrate is reabsorbed; about 56% of the filtered urea is excreted in the urine.

LOOP OF HENLE

The descending limb is relatively impermeable to solutes, but permeable to water; water is reabsorbed by osmosis. The ascending limb is impermeable to water, but relatively permeable to solutes; symporters actively transport one Na^+, one K^+, and two Cl^- from the filtrate. Leakage channels allow K^+ to recycle into the filtrate and interstitial fluid, so the overall impact of this mechanism is the reabsorption of Na^+ and Cl^-.

DISTAL CONVOLUTED TUBULE (DCT) AND COLLECTING DUCT

In the DCT and collecting duct, the reabsorption of sodium, chloride, and water continues by means of Na^+–Cl^- symporters in the apical membranes and sodium pumps in the basolateral membranes. The hormone aldosterone brings about increased sodium reabsorption by principal cells. The presence of antidiuretic hormone (ADH) increases the water permeability of principal cells, increasing the reabsorption of water. Bicarbonate ions (HCO_3^-), which are formed in the intercalated cells by the breakdown of carbonic acid, are reabsorbed.

PROXIMAL CONVOLUTED TUBULE

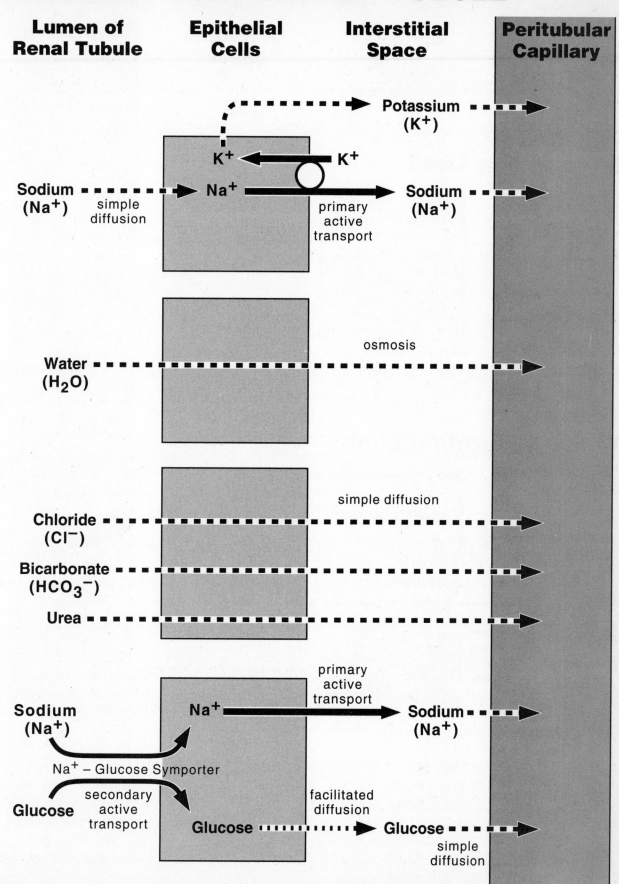

LOOP OF HENLE

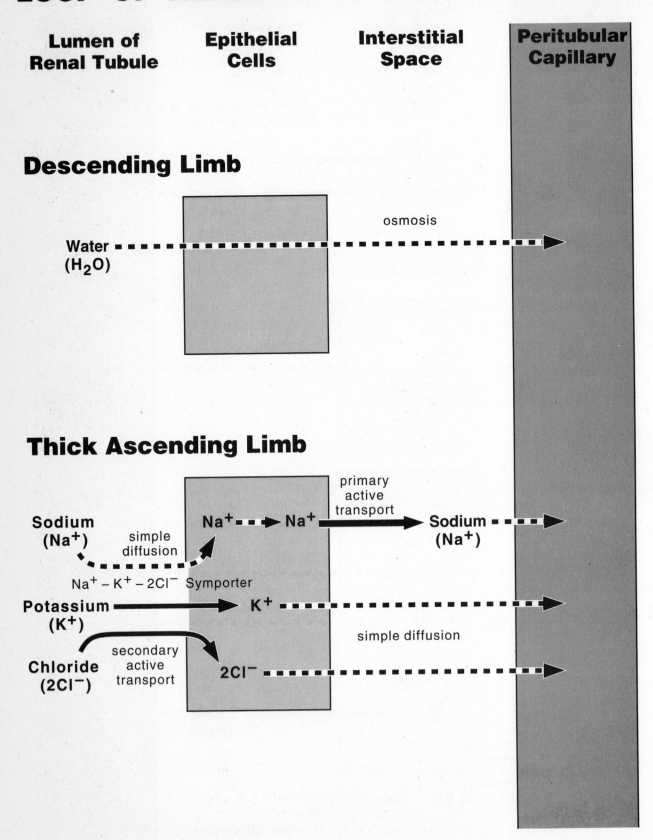

Lumen of Renal Tubule   **Epithelial Cells**   **Interstitial Space**   **Peritubular Capillary**

Descending Limb

Water (H_2O)

osmosis

Thick Ascending Limb

Sodium (Na^+)

simple diffusion

$Na^+ - K^+ - 2Cl^-$ Symporter

Potassium (K^+)

Chloride ($2Cl^-$)

secondary active transport

Na^+ Na^+

primary active transport

Sodium (Na^+)

K^+

simple diffusion

$2Cl^-$

DCT AND COLLECTING DUCTS

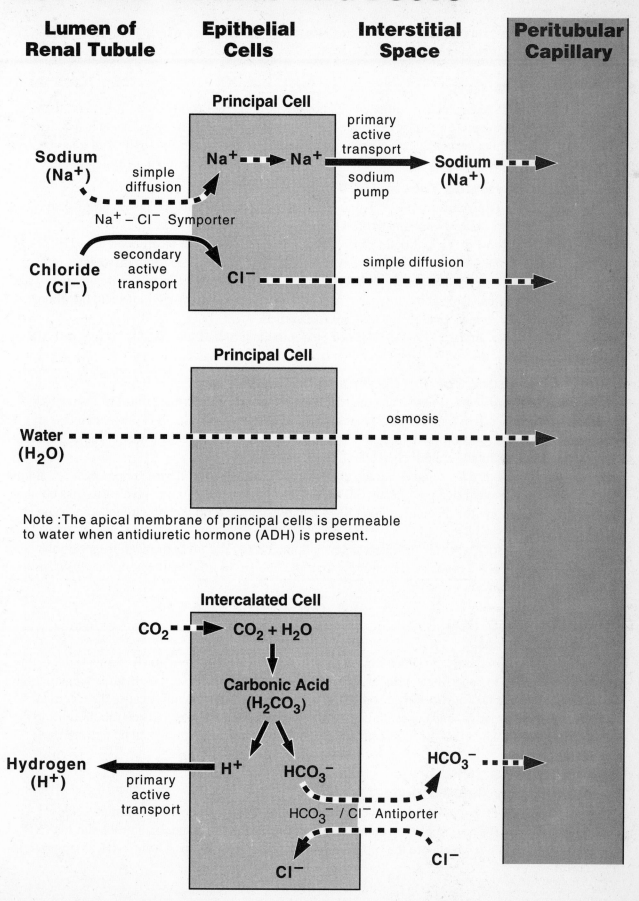

Lumen of Renal Tubule | **Epithelial Cells** | **Interstitial Space** | **Peritubular Capillary**

Principal Cell

Sodium (Na$^+$)

simple diffusion

Na$^+$ ---▶ Na$^+$

primary active transport

sodium pump

Sodium (Na$^+$)

Na$^+$ – Cl$^-$ Symporter

Chloride (Cl$^-$)

secondary active transport

Cl$^-$

simple diffusion

Principal Cell

Water (H$_2$O)

osmosis

Note : The apical membrane of principal cells is permeable to water when antidiuretic hormone (ADH) is present.

Intercalated Cell

CO$_2$ ---▶ CO$_2$ + H$_2$O

Carbonic Acid (H$_2$CO$_3$)

Hydrogen (H$^+$)

primary active transport

H$^+$

HCO$_3^-$

HCO$_3^-$

HCO$_3^-$ / Cl$^-$ Antiporter

Cl$^-$

Cl$^-$

URINE FORMATION / Tubular Secretion

Tubular Secretion Tubular secretion, the third process involved in urine formation, removes materials from the blood in the peritubular capillaries and adds them to the filtrate.

HYDROGEN IONS (H⁺)

The secretion of H⁺ takes place in epithelial cells of the PCT and collecting duct. It begins when carbon dioxide (in the presence of the enzyme carbonic anhydrase) combines with water inside an epithelial cell, forming carbonic acid. The carbonic acid then dissociates into hydrogen ions (H⁺) and bicarbonate ions (HCO_3^-). The hydrogen ions (H⁺) are secreted into the tubular fluid (filtrate).

Proximal Convoluted Tubule (PCT)

Secondary Active Transport In the PCT, the secretion of hydrogen ions (H⁺) is accomplished by secondary active transport (Na⁺/H⁺ antiporter).

Fate of the H⁺ Most of the hydrogen ions (H⁺) secreted combine with bicarbonate ions (HCO_3^-) already present in the filtrate to form carbonic acid (H_2CO_3). The carbonic acid dissociates into carbon dioxide and water. The carbon dioxide diffuses into the tubule cells, where it combines with water to form carbonic acid again; the carbonic acid dissociates into hydrogen ions and bicarbonate ions. These newly formed bicarbonate ions are reabsorbed.

Reabsorption of Na⁺ and HCO_3^- As H⁺ is secreted into the tubular fluid, HCO_3^- is reabsorbed into the blood together with Na⁺.

Distal Convoluted Tubule (DCT) and Collecting Duct

Primary Active Transport In the collecting ducts, the secretion of hydrogen ions (H⁺) is accomplished by primary active transport; the H⁺ pump (H⁺/ATP-ase) itself uses ATP and can move H⁺ against a 1000-fold concentration gradient. This occurs in intercalated cells (most of the cells in this portion of the renal tubule are principal cells).

Fate of the H⁺ Some H⁺ secreted into the collecting duct is buffered. There are two buffers, ammonia (NH_3) and monohydrogen phosphate (HPO_4^{2-}), available in the filtrate. Hydrogen ions combine with ammonia to form the ammonium ion (NH_4^+); they combine with monohydrogen phosphate to form dihydrogen phosphate ($H_2PO_4^-$). These substances are excreted in the urine.

Reabsorption of HCO_3^- Inside the intercalated cell, the HCO_3^- left over from splitting carbonic acid is transported across the basolateral membrane into the interstitial fluid by secondary active transport (HCO_3^-/Cl⁻ antiporter).

POTASSIUM IONS (K⁺)
Collecting Ducts

Electrochemical Gradient To adjust for varying dietary intake of potassium (K⁺) and to maintain homeostasis of K⁺ in body fluids, principal cells in the collecting ducts secrete a variable amount of potassium in exchange for reabsorbed sodium (Na⁺). The exchange occurs because the electrical gradient (lumen negative) and concentration gradient (higher concentration inside tubule cell) favor movement of potassium into the tubule lumen. Potassium secretion is stimulated by aldosterone.

AMMONIUM IONS (NH₄⁺)
Proximal Convoluted Tubule (PCT)

Secondary Active Transport Proximal convoluted tubule cells may deaminate amino acids to produce ammonia (NH_3). At pH 7.4, ammonia picks up a H⁺ and becomes an ammonium ion (NH_4^+). Ammonium ions are secreted into the filtrate by secondary active transport (Na⁺/NH_4^+ antiporters).

TUBULAR SECRETION

Lumen of Renal Tubule   **Epithelial Cells**

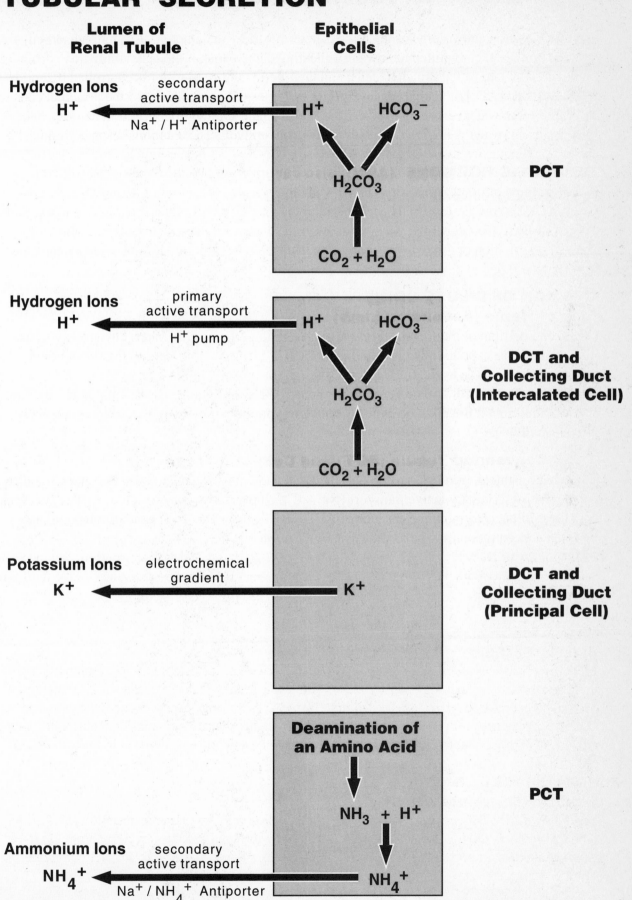

Hydrogen Ions
H^+

secondary active transport
Na^+ / H^+ Antiporter

H^+ HCO_3^-

H_2CO_3

$CO_2 + H_2O$

PCT

Hydrogen Ions
H^+

primary active transport
H^+ pump

H^+ HCO_3^-

H_2CO_3

$CO_2 + H_2O$

DCT and Collecting Duct (Intercalated Cell)

Potassium Ions
K^+

electrochemical gradient

K^+

DCT and Collecting Duct (Principal Cell)

Deamination of an Amino Acid

$NH_3 + H^+$

NH_4^+

Ammonium Ions
NH_4^+

secondary active transport
Na^+ / NH_4^+ Antiporter

PCT

URINE FORMATION / Dilute Urine

The concentration and volume of the urine is determined by the amount of water reabsorbed from the late distal convoluted tubule and collecting duct. Most of the cells lining this portion of the renal tubule are called principal cells, and their permeability to water is controlled by antidiuretic hormone (ADH). The presence of ADH increases the permeability of the principal cells to water; therefore water can be reabsorbed, forming a small volume of concentrated urine. When ADH is absent, water is not reabsorbed from the collecting ducts, so a dilute urine is formed.

ANTIDIURETIC HORMONE (ADH) also called Vasopressin

A large volume of dilute urine is produced when the plasma concentration of antidiuretic hormone (ADH) is low. A low ADH concentration means that the principal cells have a low permeability to water. Consequently, water remains in the urine as it passes through the collecting duct. The formation of dilute urine simply involves the reabsorption of more solutes than water.

FORMATION OF DILUTE URINE

Loop of Henle (Ascending Limb)

The ascending limb of the loop of Henle is relatively impermeable to water, but actively transports sodium (Na^+), potassium (K^+), and chloride (Cl^-) from the filtrate into the surrounding interstitial fluid. Thus, as the filtrate flows through this portion of the loop of Henle, its concentration drops from about 550 mOsm/liter to about 100 mOsm/liter. (When a fluid is more dilute than blood plasma it is said to be hypo-osmotic or hypotonic to blood plasma; blood plasma is 300 mOsm/liter.)

Distal Convoluted Tubule (DCT) and Collecting Duct

As the hypo-osmotic urine passes through the DCT and collecting duct, more Na^+ and Cl^- are reabsorbed by secondary active transport ($Na^+ - Cl^-$ symporters). As a result, the urine becomes even more dilute, assuming the absence of ADH. By the time the urine reaches the papillary ducts, its concentration may be as little as 65 mOsm/liter.

FORMATION OF DILUTE URINE
Plasma ADH is low.
The heavy line represents the regions that are virtually impermeable to water in the absence of antidiuretic hormone (ADH).

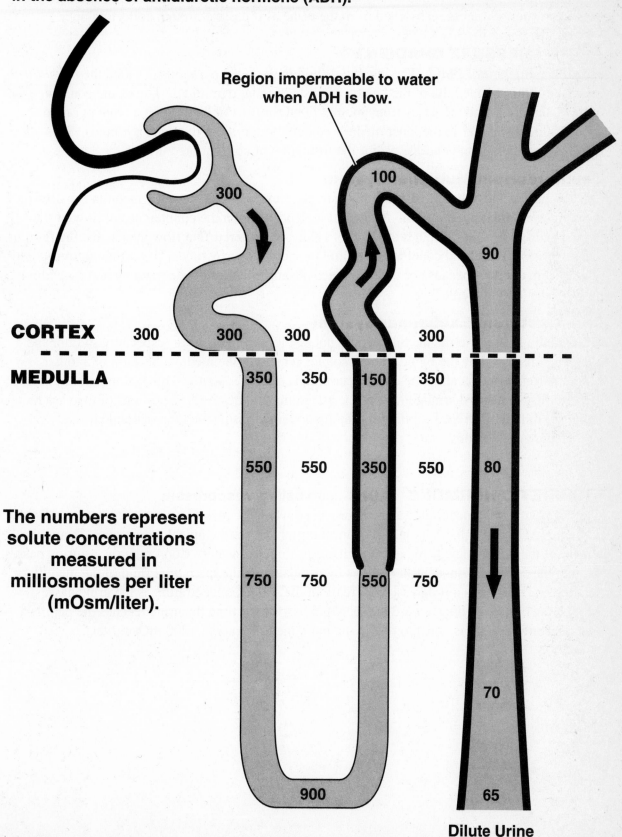

Region impermeable to water when ADH is low.

300

100

90

CORTEX　300　　300　　300　　　　300

MEDULLA　350　350　150　350

The numbers represent solute concentrations measured in milliosmoles per liter (mOsm/liter).

550　550　350　550　80

750　750　550　750

900

70

65

Dilute Urine

URINE FORMATION / Concentrated Urine

A small volume of concentrated urine is produced when the plasma concentration of antidiuretic hormone (ADH) is high. A high ADH concentration causes principal cells to have a high permeability to water. Water is reabsorbed from the urine as it passes through collecting duct.

OSMOTIC PRESSURE GRADIENT

Medullary Interstitial Fluid   The intersitial fluid in the renal pyramids is called the *medullary* interstital fluid (the medulla of the kidney consists of renal pyramids). The solute concentration of this interstitial fluid increases from about 300 mOsm/liter at the base of a renal pyramid to about 1200 mOsm/liter in the inner medulla (the tip or papilla of the renal pyramid). This osmotic pressure gradient is necessary for the formation of concentrated urine.

Countercurrent Multiplier System

The complex process that establishes this osmotic pressure gradient in the medulla is called the countercurrent multiplier system. Its operation depends upon the countercurrent flow of the tubular fluid as it passes through the loop of Henle. Countercurrent flow means that the fluid in one tube runs parallel and counter to the fluid in another nearby tube. The countercurrent multiplier system operates because of the anatomical arrangement of the descending and ascending limbs of the loop of Henle.

Countercurrent Exchanger System

The osmotic gradient in the medulla would not last long if the solutes (especially sodium and urea) were removed by the blood. These solutes remain in the medulla because of another countercurrent system called the countercurrent exchanger system.   This system operates because of the anatomical arrangement of the ascending and descending portions of the vasa recta (long, straight, loop-shaped capillaries that dip down alongside the loop of Henle in juxtamedullary nephrons).

ANTIDIURETIC HORMONE (ADH) also called Vasopressin

A small volume of concentrated urine is produced when the plasma concentration of antidiuretic hormone (ADH) is high. A high ADH concentration causes the apical membranes (facing the lumen) of the principal cells to have a high permeability to water. Consequently, as urine passes through the collecting ducts, water moves by osmosis into the interstitial fluid of the medullary pyramids. This causes a progressive increase in the solute concentration as the urine passes through the collecting duct toward the renal pelvis. By the time the urine reaches the papillary duct, its concentration is equal to that in the inner medulla (about 1200 mOsm/liter).

FORMATION OF CONCENTRATED URINE
Plasma ADH is high.
The heavy line in the thick ascending limb of the loop of Henle indicates the presence of $Na^+ - K^+ - 2Cl^-$ symporters.

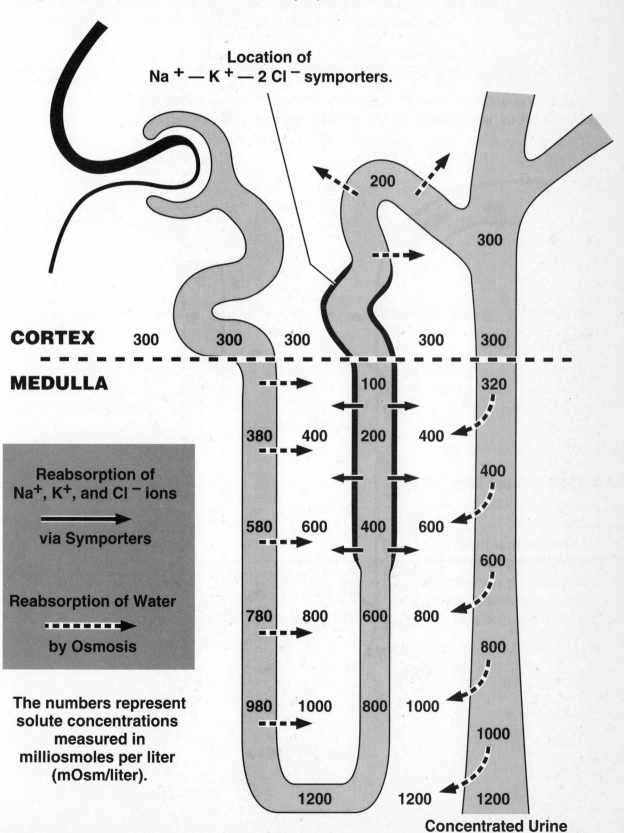

Location of $Na^+ - K^+ - 2Cl^-$ symporters.

CORTEX

MEDULLA

Reabsorption of Na^+, K^+, and Cl^- ions
via Symporters

Reabsorption of Water
by Osmosis

The numbers represent solute concentrations measured in milliosmoles per liter (mOsm/liter).

Concentrated Urine

RECYCLING OF SALTS AND UREA

The countercurrent flow of blood in the vasa recta prevents washing away of the solutes that have accumulated in the interstitial fluid of the medulla.

As blood flows down the descending portion of the vasa recta, NaCl and urea duffuse into the blood from the surrounding interstitial fluid.

As blood flows up the ascending portion of the vasa recta, NaCl and urea diffuse from the blood into the interstitial fluid.

Because of the arrangement of the ascending and descending portions of the vasa recta, solutes remain concentrated in the medulla.

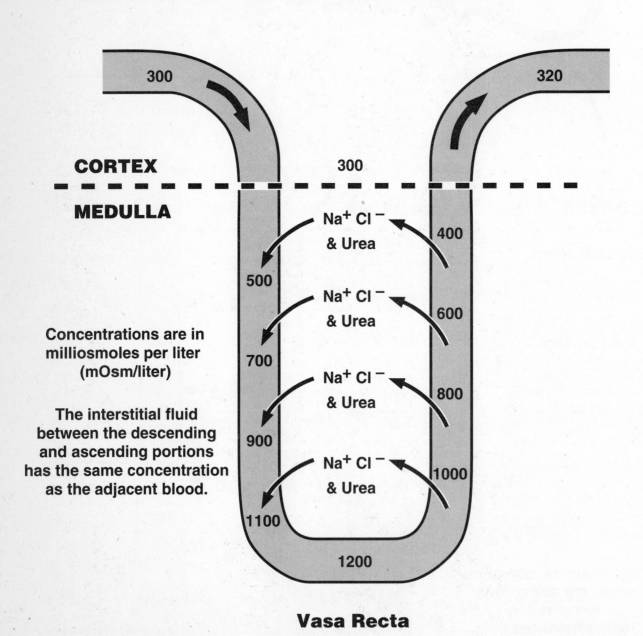

CORTEX

MEDULLA

Concentrations are in milliosmoles per liter (mOsm/liter)

The interstitial fluid between the descending and ascending portions has the same concentration as the adjacent blood.

Vasa Recta

SECRETION OF ANTIDIURETIC HORMONE

Dehydration

Blood Water Concentration Below Normal
due to
Diarrhea
Excessive Sweating
Loss of Blood

↑ **Blood Osmotic Pressure**

OSMORECEPTORS
(located in the hypothalamus)

NEUROSECRETORY CELLS
(located in the hypothalamus)

↑ **ADH production**

POSTERIOR PITUITARY

↑ **ADH secretion**

SKIN

↓ **Perspiration**

maintains blood volume
and blood pressure

KIDNEYS

↑ **H_2O reabsorption**

small volume of
concentrated urine
produced

BLOOD VESSELS

↑ **Vasoconstriction**

increases
blood pressure

43

URINE FORMATION / Urine

Water accounts for about 95% of the total volume of urine. The remaining 5% consists of solutes derived from cellular metabolism and outside sources such as drugs.

CHARACTERISTICS OF URINE

Volume   The average urine production is 1 to 2 liters daily, but the volume varies considerably.   1 liter = 1.06 quarts

Color   The color is usually yellow or amber. It varies with concentration; concentrated urine is darker in color. The color is due to urochrome, a pigment produced from the breakdown of bile. Reddish colored urine results from beets and green colored urine from asparagus. Certain diseases may affect the color; kidney stones may produce blood in the urine.

Turbidity   Turbidity refers to the degree of cloudiness. Urine is transparent when freshly voided, but becomes turbid upon standing.

Odor   Urine becomes ammonia-like upon standing. The urine of diabetics has a sweet odor due to the presence of ketone bodies.

pH   The pH ranges between 4.6 and 8.0; the average is about 6.0. The pH varies considerably with diet. High protein diets increase the acidity (lower the pH); vegetarian diets increase the alkalinity (raise the pH).

Specific Gravity   The density of urine. Specific gravity is the ratio of the weight of a volume of a substance to the weight of an equal volume of distilled water. The specific gravity of urine ranges from 1.001 to1.035. The higher the concentration of solutes, the higher the specific gravity.

SOLUTES IN URINE

Organic Solutes

Urea   Urea constitutes between 60 and 90% of all the nitrogenous waste in urine. The deamination of amino acids in the liver forms ammonia; ammonia combines with carbon dioxide to form urea, which is less toxic than ammonia.

Creatinine   Creatinine is derived primarily from the breakdown of creatine phosphate (nitrogenous substance in muscle tissues).

Uric Acid   Uric acid is a product of the catabolism of nucleic acids (DNA and RNA). It tends to crystalize and is a common component of kidney stones.

Hippuric Acid   Benzoic acid, a toxic substance present in fruits and vegetables, is converted into hippuric acid by liver cells. High-vegetable diets increase the quantity of hippuric acid excreted.

Indican   The bacterial breakdown of protein in the large intestine produces a substance called indole. It is converted into indican (a less toxic substance) by liver cells.

Ketone Bodies   Ketone bodies are substances produced during excessive triglyceride catabolism. In cases of diabetes mellitus and acute starvation, they appear in high concentrations.

Other Substances   Other substances such as carbohydrates, pigments, fatty acids, mucin, enzymes, and hormones may be present in minute quantities.

Inorganic Solutes

Cations (positive ions)   Sodium, potassium, ammonium, magnesium, and calcium.
Anions (negative ions)   Chloride, sulfate, and phosphates.

URINE
Characteristics

Volume	**1 – 2 liters (quarts) per day** (influenced by many factors)
Color	**Yellow or Amber** (varies with concentration and diet)
Turbidity	**Transparent when fresh** (becomes cloudy)
Odor	**Aromatic** (becomes ammonia-like)
pH	**Averages 6.0** (ranges between 4.6 and 8.0)
Specific Gravity	**1.001 – 1.035** (denser than water)

Organic Solutes

Nitrogenous Wastes	Urea; Creatinine; Uric Acid
Hippuric Acid	Derived from Benzoic Acid
Indican	Derived from Indole
Ketone Bodies	Derived from Triglycerides

Inorganic Solutes

Cations	Sodium; Potassium; Ammonium; Magnesium; Calcium
Anions	Chloride; Sulfate; Phosphates

3 Homeostasis

HOMEOSTASIS / Body Fluids

Body Fluid   Body water and its dissolved substances.
Solution   A mixture of substances dissolved in a liquid.
Solvent   The liquid portion of a solution.
Solute   A substance dissolved in a liquid.

FLUID COMPARTMENTS

There are three basic fluid compartments in the body: intracellular fluid, interstitial fluid, and blood plasma. The interstitial fluid and the blood plasma together constitute the extracellular fluid (ECF).

Intracellular Fluid (ICF)

About 2/3 of the fluid is within the cells and is called intracellular fluid (ICF).

Interstitial Fluid (IF)

About 75% of the extracellular fluid is outside of the cells in the tissue spaces and is called the interstitial fluid. Some of the interstitial fluid is localized in specific places such as: lymph in lymphatic vessels; cerebrospinal fluid in the brain; synovial fluid in joints; aqueous humor and vitreous body in the eyes; endolymph and perilymph in the ears; pleural, pericardial, and peritoneal fluids between serous membranes; and glomerular filtrate in the kidneys.

Blood Plasma

About 25% of the extracellular fluid is blood plasma, the fluid portion of blood.

SOLUTE CONCENTRATIONS

Osmosis is the primary method of water movement in and out of fluid compartments. So the concentration of solutes in the fluids is a major determinant of fluid balance. The following units are used to express the concentrations of solutes in body fluids.

Percent (g/dl[a] or mg/dl)   Amount of solute in a deciliter of solution.
Isotonic Saline   A 0.9% NaCl solution (0.9 g of NaCl in 100 ml of solution) is isotonic to red blood cells and is called isotonic saline. One deciliter (1/10 liter) = 100 ml.

Millimoles per Liter (mmol/liter)   Number of *millimoles* in a liter of solution.
Mole   One mole is the molecular weight of a substance expressed in grams.
Millimole   One millimole is the molecular weight of a substance expressed in milligrams.

Milliequivalents per Liter (mEq/liter)   Number of *ions* in a liter of solution.
Equivalent   One equivalent is the positive or negative charge equal to the amount of charge in one mole of hydrogen ions (H^+).
Milliequivalent   One milliequivalent is 1/1000 of an equivalent. For ions which have a single positive or negative charge, the number of mEq/liter is equal to the number of mmol/liter. For ions that have two positive or negative charges, the number of mEq/liter is twice the number of mmol/liter.

Milliosmoles per Liter (mOsm/liter)   Number of *particles* in a liter of solution.
A particle may be a whole molecule or an ion. Because it dissociates into at least two particles, an electrolyte molecule exerts a far greater effect on osmosis than a nonelectrolyte.

Osmotic Pressure (mm Hg)   Pressure required to prevent the movement of pure water through a selectively permeable membrane into a solution containing solutes.
Lower to Higher Osmotic Pressure   Water moves from an area of lower osmotic pressure (fewer particles in solution) to an area of higher osmotic pressure (more particles in solution).

FLUID COMPARTMENTS

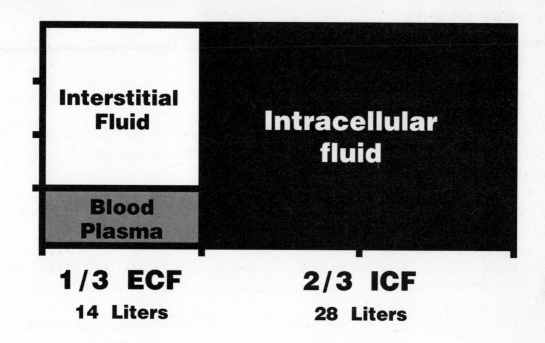

Interstitial Fluid	Intracellular fluid
Blood Plasma	

1/3 ECF
14 Liters

2/3 ICF
28 Liters

CAPILLARY BED

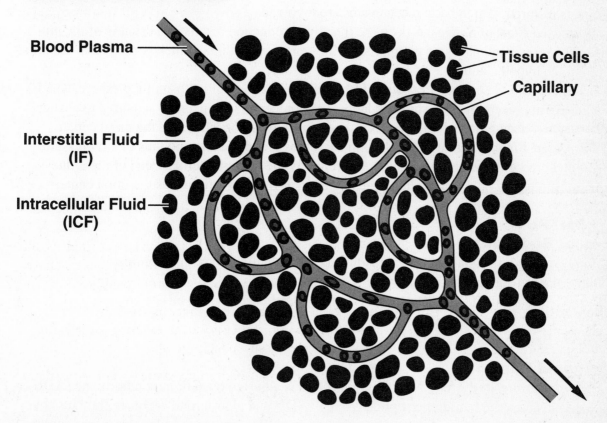

Blood Plasma

Interstitial Fluid (IF)

Intracellular Fluid (ICF)

Tissue Cells

Capillary

HOMEOSTASIS / Water Balance

PERCENT BODY WEIGHT

Water makes up from 45 to 75% of the total body weight.

Age   Infants have the greatest percentage of water, close to 75% of the total body weight. The percentage decreases with age.

Lean vs. Fat People   Since fat is basically water-free, fat people have a smaller percentage of water than lean people.

Male vs. Female   In a normal adult male, water accounts for about 60% of body weight. Since females have more subcutaneous fat than males, on average, their total body water is lower, accounting for about 55% of body weight.

FLUID INTAKE

Sources of Body Water

Daily water gain is about 2500 ml.

Preformed Water   The main source of body water is from ingested liquids (1600 ml) and foods (700 ml) that have been absorbed from the gastrointestinal tract. This water, called preformed water, amounts to about 2300 ml/day.

Metabolic Water   Another source of water is metabolic water, the water produced through deyhdration synthesis reactions (anabolism). This amounts to about 200 ml/day.

Stimulation of Thirst by Dehydration

When water loss is greater than water gain, the resulting dehydration stimulates the thirst center in the hypothalamus. The sensation of thirst is increased, fluid intake increases, and normal fluid volume is restored. Three basic mechanisms are involved:

(1) Decreased Flow of Saliva   A decrease in saliva production results in a dryness of the mucosa of the mouth and pharynx, giving rise to the sensation of thirst, which is relayed to the thirst center in the hypothalamus.

(2) Increased Blood Osmotic Pressure   Dehydration increases blood osmotic pressure, which stimulates osmoreceptors in the hypothalamus (osmoreceptors are neurons sensitive to changes in the water concentration of body fluids). These osmoreceptors stimulate the thirst center.

(3) Decreased Blood Volume   Dehydration decreases blood volume and thus blood pressure. Low blood pressure stimulates the release of renin by the juxtaglomerular cells of the kidneys. Renin promotes activation of the hormone angiotensin II, which stimulates the thirst center.

FLUID OUTPUT

Loss of Body Water

Normally, water loss equals water gain, so the body maintains a constant volume.

Kidneys   Excrete about 1500 ml/day.

Skin   Excretes about 500 ml/day (evaporation = 400ml; sweat = 100 ml).

Lungs   Excrete about 300 ml/day.

GI Tract   Excretes about 200 ml/day.

Hormonal Control

ADH, Aldosterone, and ANP   Normally, fluid loss is adjusted by antidiuretic hormone (ADH), aldosterone, and atrial natriuretic peptide (ANP). ADH and aldosterone *decrease* fluid loss by stimulating the reabsorption of water in the kidneys; ANP *increases* fluid loss by increasing the volume of urine excreted. Under abnormal conditions, other factors may influence fluid loss.

FLUID INTAKE AND OUTPUT

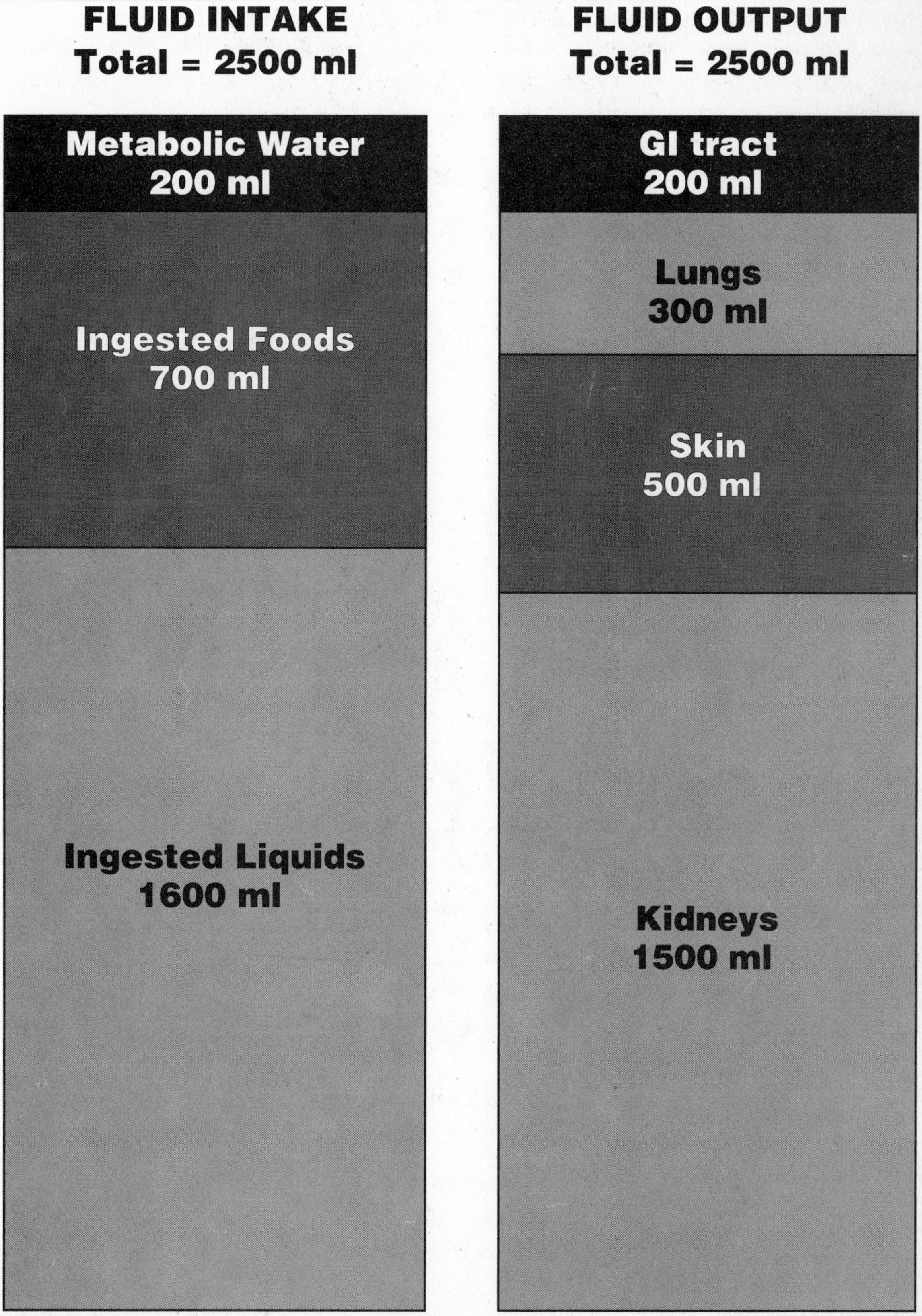

FLUID INTAKE
Total = 2500 ml

- Metabolic Water 200 ml
- Ingested Foods 700 ml
- Ingested Liquids 1600 ml

FLUID OUTPUT
Total = 2500 ml

- GI tract 200 ml
- Lungs 300 ml
- Skin 500 ml
- Kidneys 1500 ml

FACTORS THAT STIMULATE THIRST

Dehydration stimulates thirst in at least three ways :
(1) A decrease in saliva production leads to dryness of the mouth and pharynx.
(2) An increase in blood osmotic pressure stimulates osmoreceptors.
(3) A decrease in blood volume and blood pressure stimulates the release of renin.

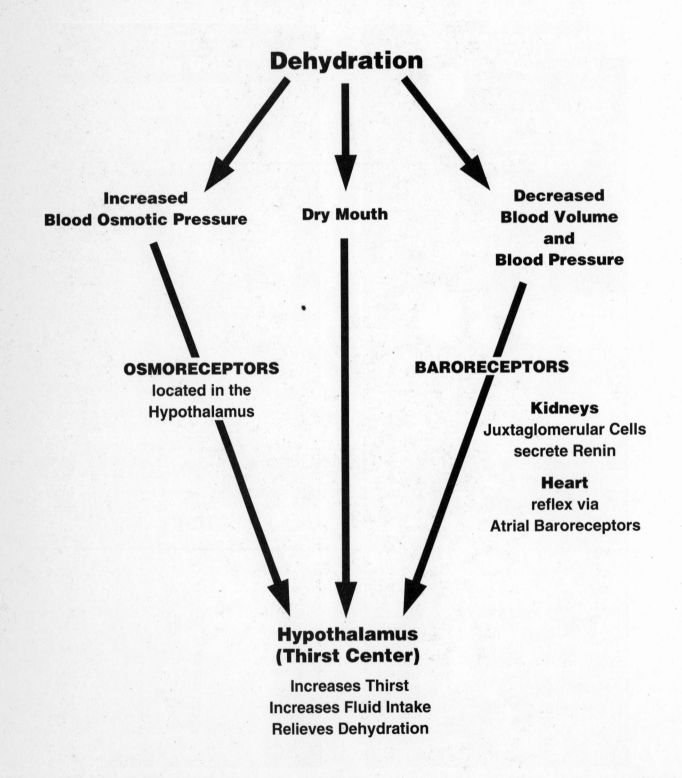

Dehydration

Increased
Blood Osmotic Pressure

Dry Mouth

Decreased
Blood Volume
and
Blood Pressure

OSMORECEPTORS
located in the
Hypothalamus

BARORECEPTORS

Kidneys
Juxtaglomerular Cells
secrete Renin

Heart
reflex via
Atrial Baroreceptors

Hypothalamus
(Thirst Center)

Increases Thirst
Increases Fluid Intake
Relieves Dehydration

ANTIDIURETIC HORMONE

Antidiuretic hormone (ADH) causes the principal cells of the distal DCT and collecting ducts to be permeable to water.

Water loss or gain that is out of proportion to sodium loss or gain causes a change in the osmolarity of body fluids.

The receptors that monitor changes in the osmolarity of body fluids are called osmoreceptors and are located in the hypothalamus.
They initiate the reflexes controlling ADH secretion.

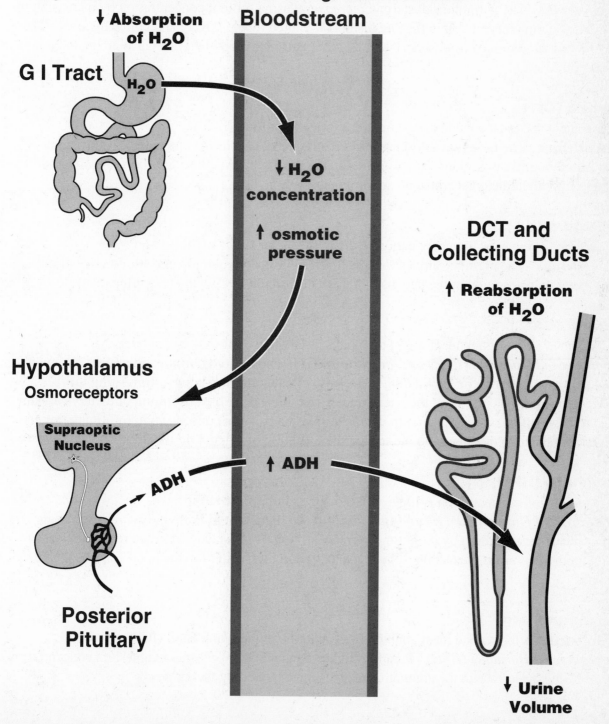

↓ Absorption of H_2O

Bloodstream

G I Tract

H_2O

↓ H_2O concentration

↑ osmotic pressure

DCT and Collecting Ducts

↑ Reabsorption of H_2O

Hypothalamus
Osmoreceptors

Supraoptic Nucleus

↑ ADH

ADH

Posterior Pituitary

↓ Urine Volume

HOMEOSTASIS / Electrolyte Balance

Electrolytes   Many solutes in body fluids are electrolytes—compounds that dissociate into ions.
Ion   Any particle that has an electrical charge (positive or negative).
Cation   A positively charged ion.
Anion   A negatively charged ion.

Sodium (Na$^+$)

Sodium is the most abundant ion in the extracellular fluid (ECF).
Aldosterone   The hormone aldosterone *increases* plasma sodium concentration by increasing the rate of sodium reabsorption in the late distal convoluted tubule (DCT) and collecting duct. The hormones antidiuretic hormone (ADH) and atrial natriuetic peptide (ANP) also affect sodium concentrations.

Chloride (Cl$^-$)

Chloride is the most abundant anion in the extracellular fluid (ECF).
Aldosterone   The hormone aldosterone indirectly *increases* plasma chloride concentration. Aldosterone increases sodium reabsorption in the renal tubules; chloride follows passively down the electrical gradient generated by sodium reabsorption.

Potassium (K$^+$)

Potassium is the most abundant cation in the intracellular fluid (ICF).
Aldosterone   The hormone aldosterone *decreases* plasma potassium concentration by stimulating potassium secretion in the late distal convoluted tubule (DCT) and collecting duct.

Calcium (Ca^{2+})

Calcium is the most abundant ion in the body. A large amount is stored in bones.
Parathyroid Hormone (PTH) and Calcitonin (CT)   Parathyroid hormone *increases* plasma calcium concentration by stimulating the release of calcium from bones, stimulating the reabsorption of calcium from the renal tubules, and increasing the absorption of dietary calcium from the small intestine. Calcitonin *decreases* plasma calcium concentration by stimulating the uptake of calcium by bones and increasing the excretion of calcium in the urine.

Phosphate (HPO$_4^{2-}$)

Phosphate ion concentration is highest in the intracellular fluid (ICF).
Parathyroid Hormone (PTH) and Calcitonin (CT)   Parathyroid hormone *decreases* plasma phosphate concentration by inhibiting the reabsorption of phosphate from the renal tubules. Calcitonin *decreases* plasma phosphate concentration by stimulating the uptake of phosphate by bones.

Magnesium (Mg^{2+})

Magnesium is the second most abundant cation in the intracellular fluid (ICF).
Parathyroid Hormone (PTH)   Parathyroid hormone *increases* plasma magnesium concentration by causing a decrease in the amount of magnesium excreted by the kidneys.

ELECTROLYTE CONCENTRATIONS
Relative Concentrations of the Major Electrolytes (ions)

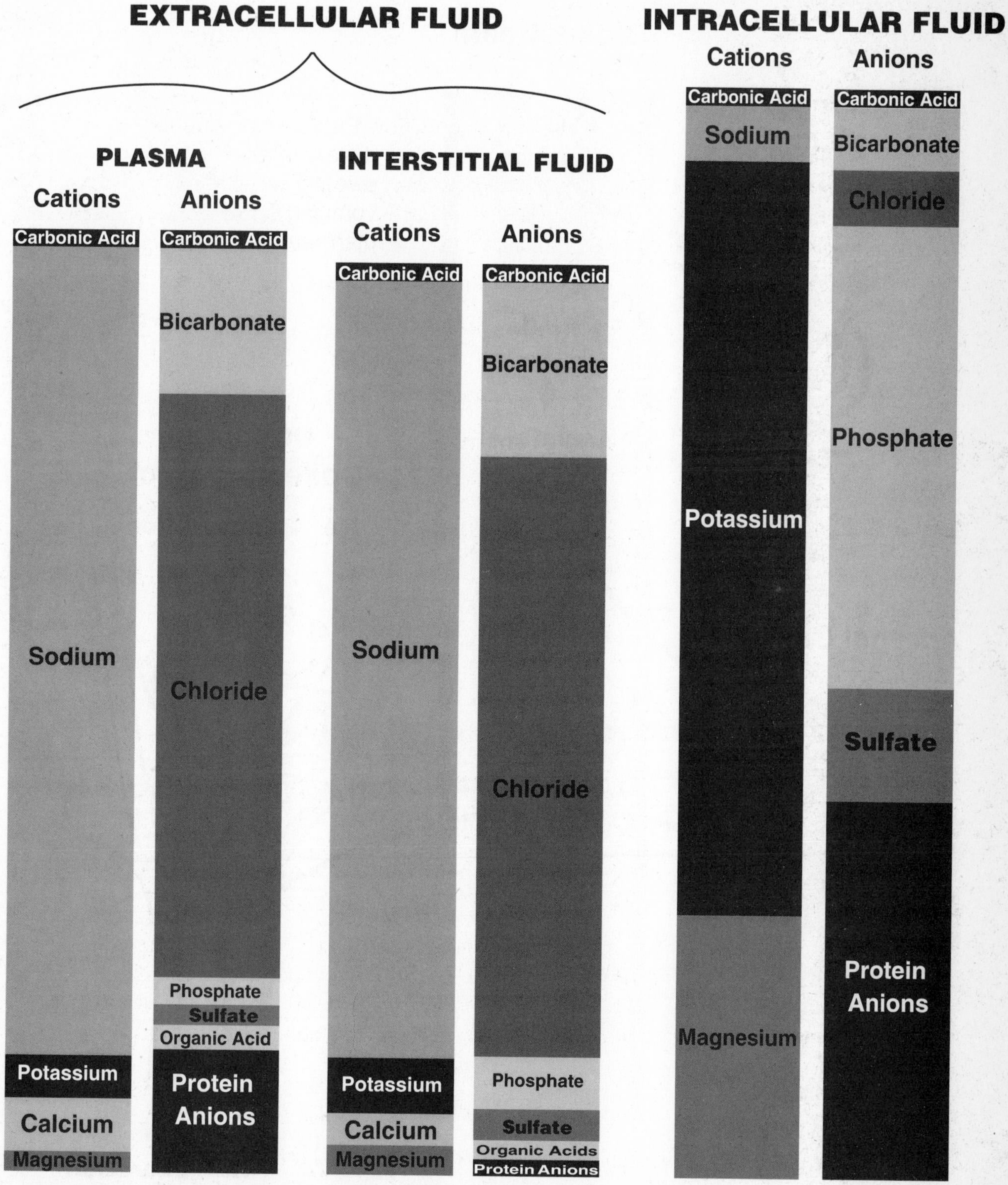

EXTRACELLULAR FLUID

PLASMA

Cations | Anions

Carbonic Acid | Carbonic Acid

Bicarbonate

Sodium

Chloride

Phosphate
Sulfate
Organic Acid

Potassium | Protein Anions

Calcium

Magnesium

INTERSTITIAL FLUID

Cations | Anions

Carbonic Acid | Carbonic Acid

Bicarbonate

Sodium

Chloride

Potassium | Phosphate

Calcium | Sulfate
Organic Acids
Magnesium | Protein Anions

INTRACELLULAR FLUID

Cations | Anions

Carbonic Acid | Carbonic Acid

Sodium | Bicarbonate

Chloride

Potassium | Phosphate

Sulfate

Magnesium | Protein Anions

SODIUM BALANCE

Aldosterone <u>increases</u> the plasma sodium (Na$^+$) concentration by increasing the rate of Na$^+$ reabsorption in the DCT and collecting ducts.

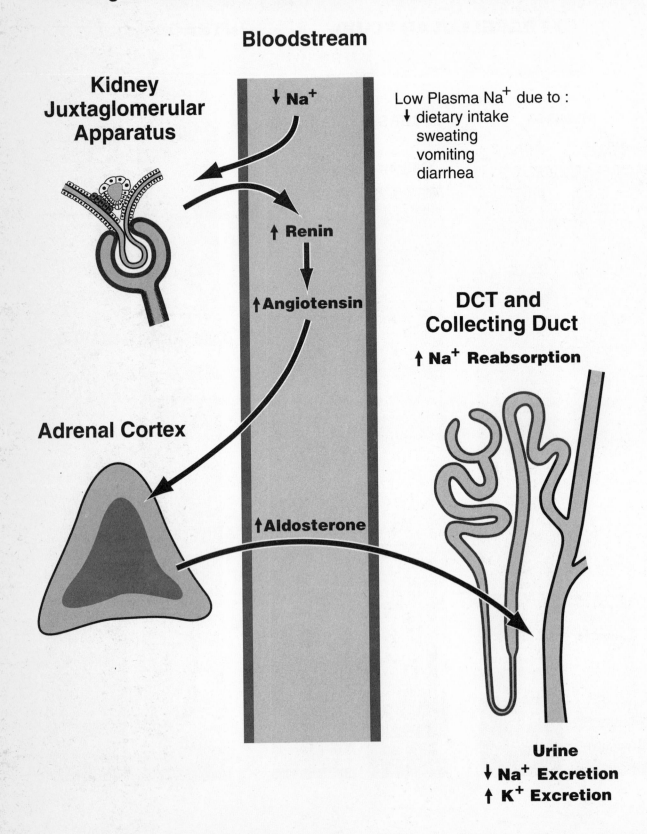

Bloodstream

Kidney Juxtaglomerular Apparatus

↓ Na$^+$

Low Plasma Na$^+$ due to :
↓ dietary intake
   sweating
   vomiting
   diarrhea

↑ Renin

↑ Angiotensin

DCT and Collecting Duct

↑ Na$^+$ Reabsorption

Adrenal Cortex

↑ Aldosterone

Urine
↓ Na$^+$ Excretion
↑ K$^+$ Excretion

POTASSIUM BALANCE

Aldosterone <u>decreases</u> the plasma potassium (K^+) concentration by increasing the rate of K^+ secretion in the DCT and collecting ducts.

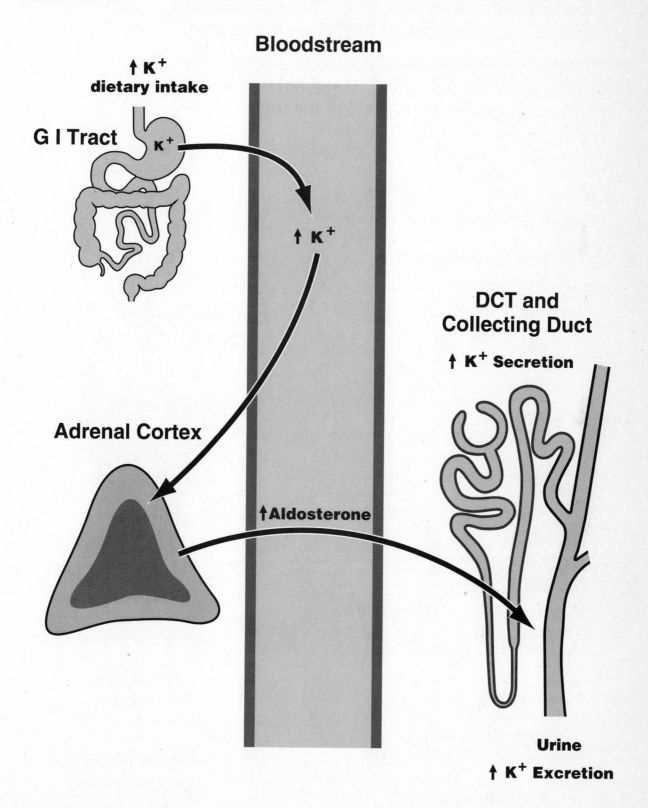

CALCIUM BALANCE

Parathyroid hormone (PTH) <u>increases</u> plasma calcium concentration by :
(1) stimulating the release of Ca^{2+} (calcium) from bones;
(2) stimulating the reabsorption of Ca^{2+} in renal tubules;
(3) increasing the absorption of Ca^{2+} from the GI tract.

Calcitonin (CT) <u>decreases</u> plasma calcium concentration by :
(1) stimulating the uptake of Ca^{2+} (calcium) by bones;
(2) increasing the excretion of Ca^{2+} in the urine.

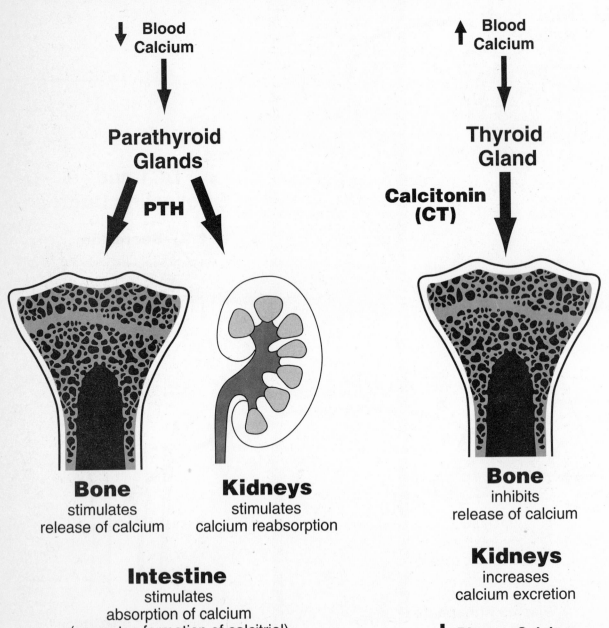

↓ Blood Calcium

Parathyroid Glands

PTH

↑ Blood Calcium

Thyroid Gland

Calcitonin (CT)

Bone
stimulates
release of calcium

Kidneys
stimulates
calcium reabsorption

Intestine
stimulates
absorption of calcium
(promotes formation of calcitriol)

↑ Plasma Calcium

Bone
inhibits
release of calcium

Kidneys
increases
calcium excretion

↓ Plasma Calcium

PHOSPHATE BALANCE

PTH <u>decreases</u> plasma phosphate (HPO_4^{2-}) concentration by inhibiting the reabsorption of HPO_4^{2-} in renal tubules.

CT <u>decreases</u> plasma phosphate (HPO_4^{2-}) concentration by stimulating the uptake of HPO_4^{2-} by bones.

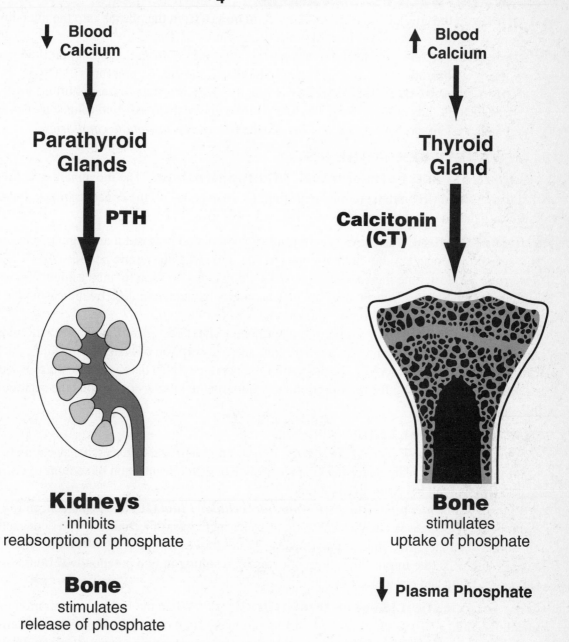

↓ Blood Calcium

↑ Blood Calcium

Parathyroid Glands

Thyroid Gland

PTH

Calcitonin (CT)

Kidneys
inhibits
reabsorption of phosphate

Bone
stimulates
uptake of phosphate

Bone
stimulates
release of phosphate

↓ Plasma Phosphate

↓ Plasma Phosphate

note :
in response to PTH, more phosphate is
lost in the urine than is gained from bones.

HOMEOSTASIS / Movement of Body Fluids

The main fluid compartments in the body are the *blood plasma, interstitial fluid (IF),* and *intracellular fluid (ICF).* Although fluids are in constant motion from one compartment to another, the volume of fluid in each compartment remains fairly stable. Water moves in and out of fluid compartments by osmosis, and osmotic pressure gradients are determined by solute concentrations (electrolytes).

MOVEMENT BETWEEN PLASMA AND IF

Filtration At the arterial end of a capillary, fluid moves from the plasma into the interstitial fluid by filtration; the driving force is blood hydrostatic pressure (BHP).

Reabsorption At the venule end of a capillary, fluid moves from the interstitial fluid back into the plasma by reabsorption; the driving force is blood colloid osmotic pressure (BCOP).

Starling's Law of the Capillaries Normally, there is a state of near equilibrium at the arterial and venous ends of a capillary: the filtered fluid and reabsorbed fluid (plus that picked up by the lymphatic system) are nearly equal. This is called *Starling's law of the capillaries.*

MOVEMENT BETWEEN IF AND ICF

Sodium (Na^+) and Potassium (K^+) Concentrations The movement of fluid between the interstitial fluid (IF) and the intracellular fluid (ICF) depends on the concentrations of sodium and potassium. They determine the net flow of water by osmosis.

Hormonal Control Plasma concentrations of sodium and potassium are regulated by three hormones: aldosterone, antidiuretic hormone (ADH), and atrial natriuretic peptide (ANP).

Aldosterone Aldosterone *increases* the plasma sodium concentration by increasing the reabsorption of sodium by the kidneys; it *decreases* the plasma potassium concentration by increasing the rate of potassium secetion (and excretion) by the kidneys.

Antidiuretic Hormone (ADH) Antidiuretic hormone (ADH) *decreases* the plasma sodium and potassium concentrations indirectly by increasing the reabsorption of water by the kidneys.

Atrial Natriuretic Peptide (ANP) Atrial natriuretic peptide (ANP) *decreases* the plasma sodium concentration by inhibiting the reabsorption of sodium by the kidneys (it inhibits the secretion of renin and aldosterone).

ELECTROLYTE IMBALANCE

Vomiting, Diarrhea, or Excessive Sweating If vomiting, diarrhea, or excessive sweating is followed by the intake of plain water (lacking electrolytes), the concentration of sodium in the interstitial fluid (IF) can fall below the normal range.

Net Osmosis from Interstitial Fluid (IF) into Intracellular Fluid (ICF) As the concentration of sodium in the IF decreases, the concentration of water increases; this creates a water concentration gradient between these two fluid compartments. Water moves from the hypo-osmotic interstitial fluid (IF) into cells (the intracellular fluid or cytosol), resulting in two potentially serious conditions: water intoxication and circulatory shock.

Water Intoxication (Severe Overhydration) When the water concentration in the intracellular fluid (ICF) is above normal, the condition is called overhydration. Severe overhydration is called water intoxication; it produces neurological symptoms ranging from disoriented behavior to convulsions, coma, and even death.

Circulatory Shock Circulatory shock is a condition that results from low blood pressure caused by a loss of blood volume. The movement of water from the interstital fluid (IF) into the intracellular fluid (ICF) lowers the water concentration of the IF. This generates a water concentration gradient between the plasma and the IF. Water moves out of the plasma into the IF, causing a loss of blood volume that may lead to circulatory shock.

ELECTROLYTE IMBALANCE

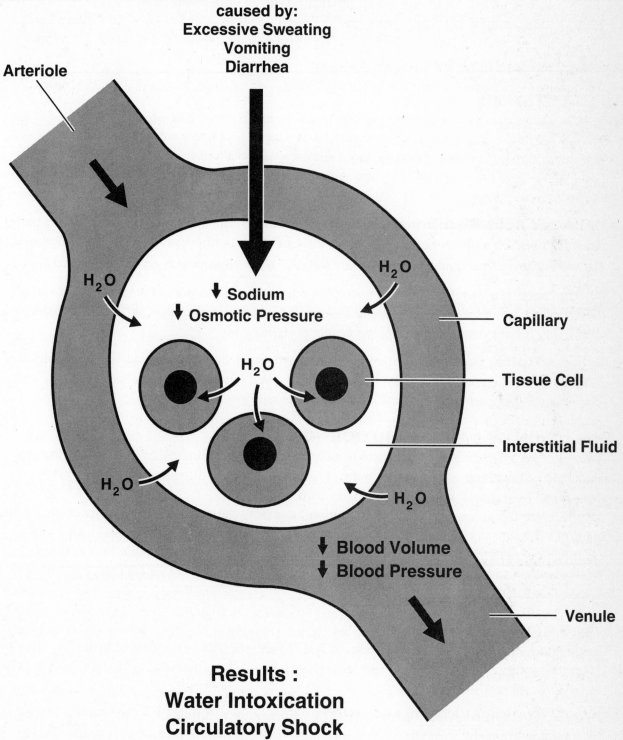

Loss of Electrolytes
caused by:
Excessive Sweating
Vomiting
Diarrhea

Arteriole

H_2O

H_2O

⬇ Sodium
⬇ Osmotic Pressure

H_2O

H_2O

H_2O

Capillary

Tissue Cell

Interstitial Fluid

H_2O

H_2O

⬇ Blood Volume
⬇ Blood Pressure

Venule

Results :
Water Intoxication
Circulatory Shock

HOMEOSTASIS / Acid–Base Balance

The acid–base balance of the body is maintained by controlling the hydrogen ion (H^+) concentration of body fluids, especially the extracellular fluid (ECF). The maintenance of the H^+ concentration within a narrow pH range (between 7.35 and 7.45) is essential to survival. Hydrogen ion homeostasis depends on three homeostatic mechanisms: buffer systems, exhalation of carbon dioxide, and kidney regulation of pH.

BUFFER SYSTEMS

Buffer systems act quickly (within fractions of a second) to prevent rapid, drastic changes in the pH of body fluids. Most buffer systems consist of a weak acid and a weak base. When there is an excess of hydrogen ions, the weak base combines with the hydrogen ions, forming a weak acid. When there is a shortage of hydrogen ions, the weak acid dissociates, releasing more hydrogen ions.

Carbonic Acid–Bicarbonate Buffer System   The carbonic acid–bicarbonate buffer system is the most abundant buffer system in the ECF; it is an important regulator of blood pH. The weak base in this system is *bicarbonate* (HCO_3^-); the weak acid is *carbonic acid* (H_2CO_3).

Phosphate Buffer System   Phosphates are important buffers in the intracellular fluid (inside cells) and in the urine. The weak base in this system is called *monohydrogen phosphate* (HPO_4^{2-}); the weak acid is *dihydrogen phosphate* ($H_2PO_4^-$).

Protein Buffer System   Proteins are the most abundant buffers in body cells and blood. Hemoglobin (inside red blood cells) is an especially good buffer. The weak base in this system is the *amine group* ($-NH_2$); the weak acid is the *carboxyl group* ($-COOH$).

EXHALATION OF CARBON DIOXIDE (CO_2)

The pH of body fluids may be adjusted, usually in one to three minutes, by a change in the rate and depth of breathing. An increase in the exhalation of carbon dioxide increases the pH; a decrease in the exhalation of carbon dioxide decreases the pH.

When the blood hydrogen ion concentration increases, chemoreceptors in the medulla oblongata (of the brainstem) are activated. They stimulate the inspiratory center (also located in the medulla oblongata). The inspiratory center sends nerve impulses to the respiratory muscles, which contract more forcefully and with greater frequency; this increases the exhalation of carbon dioxide.

KIDNEY REGULATION OF pH

Renal tubules may raise blood pH in three ways: (1) secretion and excretion of hydrogen ions; (2) reabsorption of filtered bicarbonate ions (HCO_3^-); and (3) synthesis and absorption of newly formed bicarbonate ions.

Proximal Convoluted Tubule (PCT)   Epithelial cells lining the PCT secrete hydrogen ions into the filtrate by secondary active transport. Filtered bicarbonate ions are reabsorbed by diffusion.

Distal Convoluted Tubule (DCT) and Collecting Ducts   Intercalated cells of the DCT and collecting duct secrete hydrogen into the filtrate by primary active transport. Bicarbonate ions synthesized in the intercalated cells are absorbed by secondary active transport.

BUFFER SYSTEMS

Carbonic Acid–Bicarbonate Buffer System

Excess H$^+$ a weak base (bicarbonate) combines with H$^+$

$$HCO_3^- + \boxed{H^+} \longrightarrow H_2CO_3 \longrightarrow H_2O + CO_2$$

Shortage of H$^+$ a weak acid (carbonic acid) dissociates, releasing H$^+$

$$H_2CO_3 \longrightarrow \boxed{H^+} + HCO_3^-$$

Phosphate Buffer System

Excess H$^+$ a weak base (monohydrogen phosphate) combines with H$^+$

$$HPO_4^{2-} + \boxed{H^+} \longrightarrow H_2PO_4^-$$

Shortage of H$^+$ a weak acid (dihydrogen phosphate) dissociates, releasing H$^+$

$$H_2PO_4^- \longrightarrow \boxed{H^+} + HPO_4^{2-}$$

Protein Buffer System

Excess H$^+$ a weak base (amine group) combines with H$^+$

$$\begin{matrix} & & R & \\ & & | & \\ H{>}N- & C & -COOH \\ H & & | & \\ & & H & \end{matrix} + \boxed{H^+} \longrightarrow \begin{matrix} & H & R & \\ & | & | & \\ \boxed{H^+}-N- & C & -COOH \\ & | & | & \\ & H & H & \end{matrix}$$

Shortage of H$^+$ a weak acid (carboxyl group) dissociates, releasing H$^+$

$$\begin{matrix} & R & \\ & | & \\ H{>}N-C{-}(COOH) \\ H & | & \\ & H & \end{matrix} \longrightarrow \boxed{H^+} + \begin{matrix} & R & \\ & | & \\ H{>}N-C-COO^- \\ H & | & \\ & H & \end{matrix}$$

EXHALATION OF CARBON DIOXIDE

The pH of body fluids may be adjusted by a change in the rate and depth of breathing.

BLOOD

 Blood H⁺ Concentration

High blood CO_2 concentration
leads to high H_2CO_3 concentration
and high hydrogen ion concentration
(low pH)

CHEMORECEPTORS

(located in the medulla oblongata)

Activated by H⁺
Stimulate the Inspiratory Center

INSPIRATORY CENTER

(located in medulla oblongata)

Sends nerve impulses to
the Respiratory Muscles

RESPIRATORY MUSCLES

↑ **Rate and Depth
of Breathing**

LUNGS

↑ **Exhalation of CO_2**

BLOOD

↓ **Blood H⁺ Concentration**

Lower blood CO_2 concentration
leads to lower H_2CO_3 concentration
and lower hydrogen ion concentration
(normal pH)

EXCRETION OF HYDROGEN IONS

Renal tubules may raise blood pH in three ways :
(1) Secretion (and excretion) of H^+.
(2) Reabsorption of filtered HCO_3^-.
(3) Synthesis and absorption of newly formed HCO_3^-.

In the PCT, H^+ ions are secreted by secondary active transport; HCO_3^- is reabsorbed by diffusion. Although the reabsorbed HCO_3^- and the filtered HCO_3^- are of different origins, filtered HCO_3^- disappears at the same time that the HCO_3^- formed in the cell enters the blood; so the net effect is the reabsorption of the filtered bicarbonate.

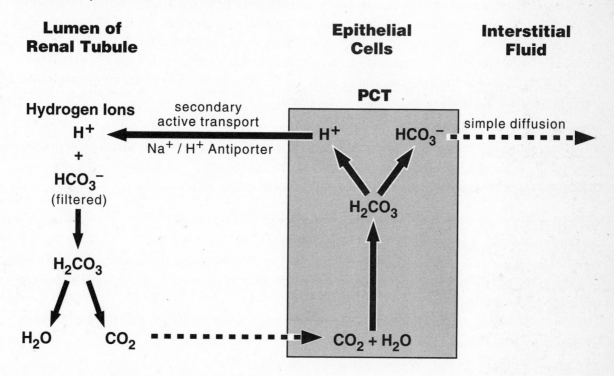

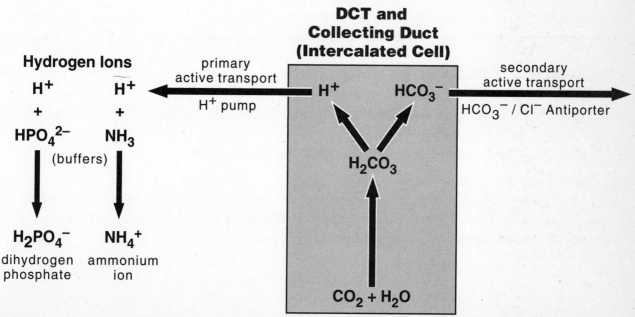

HOMEOSTASIS / Acid–Base Imbalances

ACIDOSIS AND ALKALOSIS

Normal Blood pH   The normal blood pH is 7.35 to 7.45.

Acidosis (Acidemia)   Acidosis is a condition in which blood pH is below 7.35.

Alkalosis (Alkalemia)   Alkalosis is a condition in which blood pH is higher than 7.45.

Carbon Dioxide Partial Pressure (pCO_2)   The concentration of carbon dioxide in plasma.

Compensation

Compensation   Compensation is the physiological response to an acid-base imbalance.

Respiratory Compensation   If a person has an altered pH due to metabolic causes, respiratory mechanisms (hyperventilation or hypoventilation) can help compensate for the alteration. Respiratory compensation occurs within minutes and is maximized within hours.

Metabolic Compensation   If a person has an altered pH due to respiratory causes, metabolic mechanisms (kidney excretion) can compensate for the alteration. Metabolic compensation may begin in minutes but takes days to reach a maximum.

Physiological Effects

The principal physiological effect of acidosis is depression of the central nervous system through depression of synaptic transmission. If the blood pH falls below 7, depression of the nervous system is so severe that the individual becomes comatose and dies.

RESPIRATORY ACIDOSIS AND ALKALOSIS

Acidosis (arterial blood pCO_2 is above 45 mm Hg)

Respiratory acidosis is characterized by an elevated pCO_2 of arterial blood. A buildup of carbon dioxide in the blood leads to an increase in the production of carbonic acid, which dissociates releasing hydrogen ions.

Metabolic Compensation   The kidneys attempt to compensate by *increasing* the excretion of hydrogen ions and by *increasing* the reabsorption of bicarbonate ions.

Alkalosis (arterial blood pCO_2 is below 35 mm Hg)

In respiratory alkalosis the arterial blood pCO_2 is decreased. Hyperventilation increases the exhalation of carbon dioxide, causing the pH to increase.

Metabolic Compensation   The kidneys attempt to compensate by *decreasing* the excretion of hydrogen ions and *decreasing* the reabsorption of bicarbonate ions.

METABOLIC ACIDOSIS AND ALKALOSIS

Acidosis (bicarbonate ion concentration is below 22 mEq/liter)

In metabolic acidosis there is a decrease in bicarbonate ion concentration. The decrease in pH is caused by loss of bicarbonate.

Respiratory Compensation   Compensation is by hyperventilation.

Alkalosis (bicarbonate ion concentration is above 26 mEq/liter)

In metabolic alkalosis there is an increase in the bicarbonate ion concentration. A nonrespiratory loss of acid by the body or excessive intake of alkaline drugs causes the pH to increase.

Respiratory Compensation   Compensation is by hypoventilation.

ACIDOSIS AND ALKALOSIS
Acidosis (pH below 7.35)

Respiratory Acidosis

Definition : $p\,CO_2$ above 45 mm Hg

Cause : hypoventilation

Compensation : increased excretion of H^+
increased reabsorption of HCO_3^-

Metabolic Acidosis

Definition : HCO_3^- below 22 mEq/liter

Cause : loss of bicarbonate (diarrhea; ketosis; renal dysfunction)

Compensation : hyperventilation

Alkalosis (pH above 7.45)

Respiratory Alkalosis

Definition : $p\,CO_2$ below 35 mm Hg

Cause : hyperventilation

Compensation : decreased excretion of H^+
decreased reabsorption of HCO_3^-

Metabolic Alkalosis

Definition : HCO_3^- above 26 mEq/liter

Cause : loss of acid (vomiting; diuretics; alkaline drugs)

Compensation : hypoventilation

Part II : Self-Testing Exercises

Unlabeled illustrations from Part I

URINARY SYSTEM

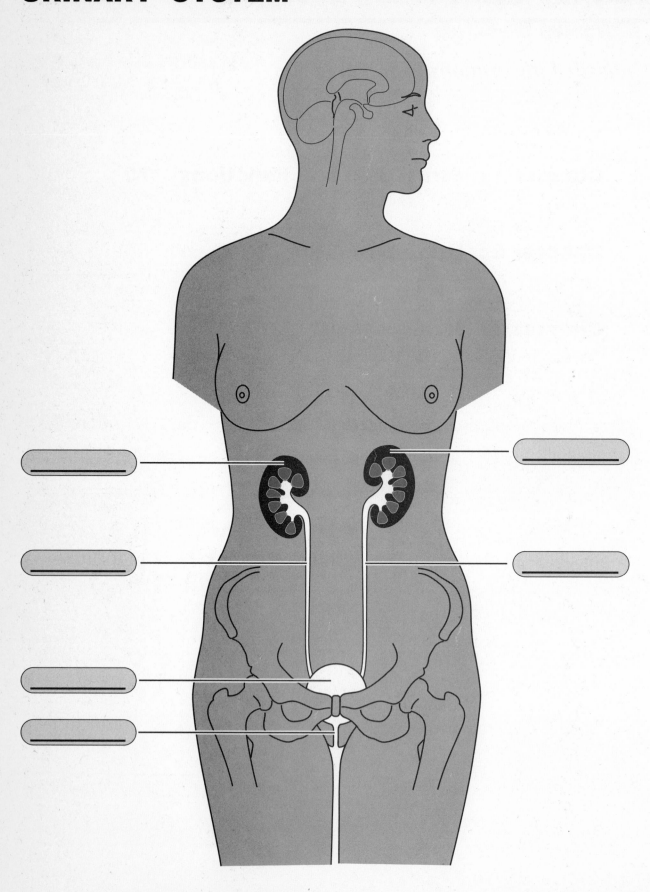

RIGHT KIDNEY
Coronal Section

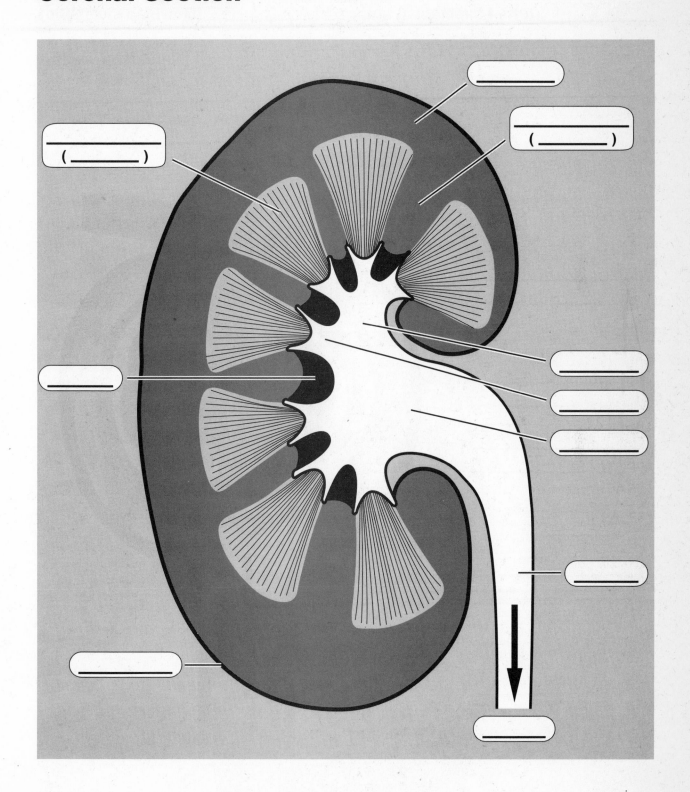

RENAL CORPUSCLE

The renal corpuscle has two components :
_____ (tuft of capillaries) and _____ (Bowman's capsule).

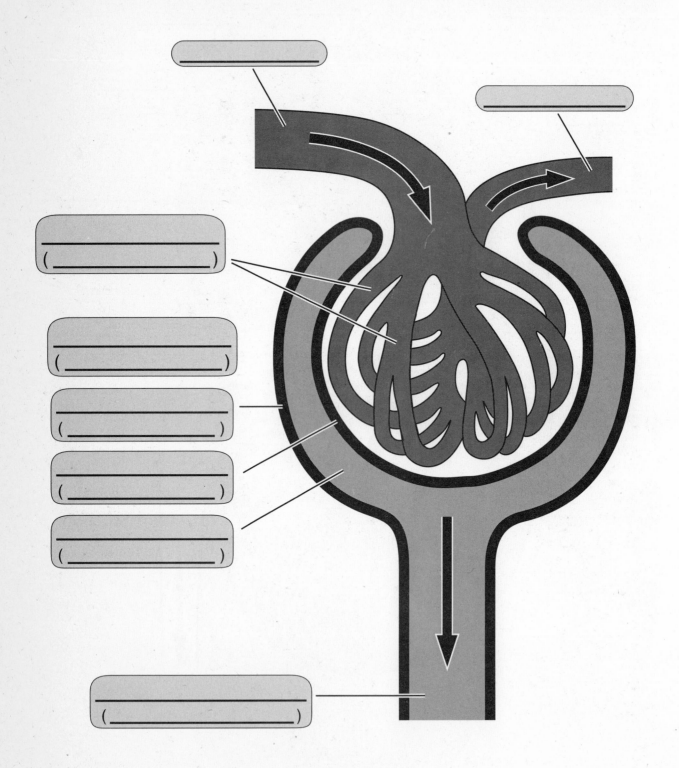

CORTICAL NEPHRON

Location

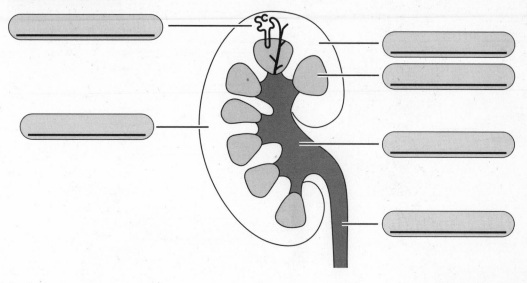

Parts

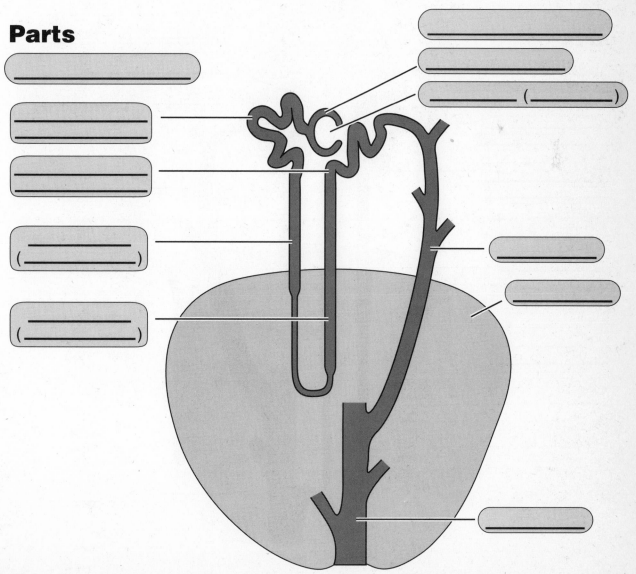

JUXTAMEDULLARY NEPHRON

Location

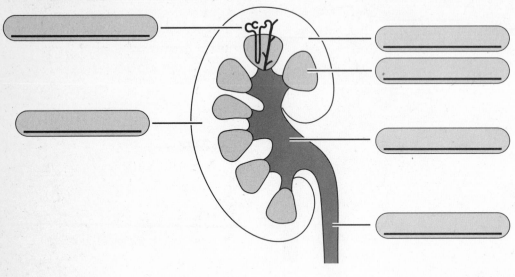

Parts

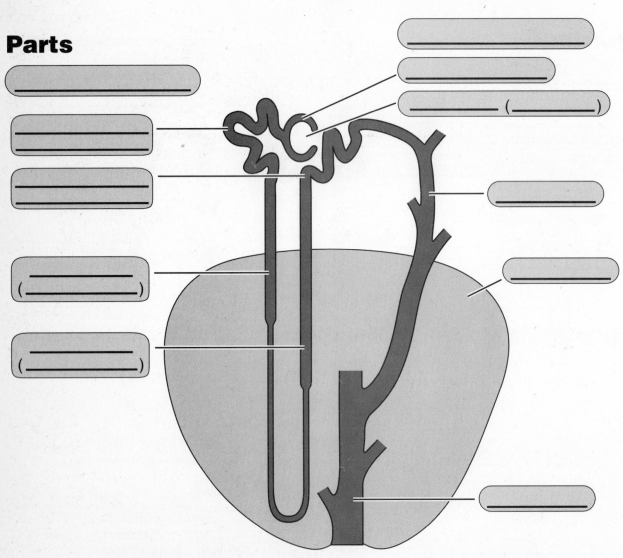

ENDOTHELIAL – CAPSULAR MEMBRANE

Renal Corpuscle

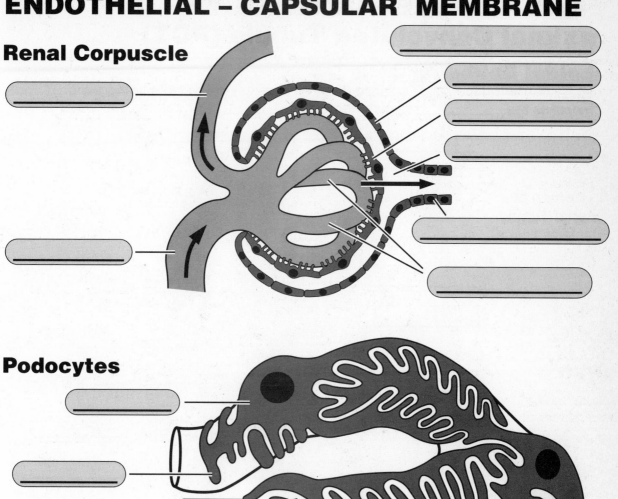

Podocytes

Endothelial–Capsular Membrane

LUMEN OF
GLOMERULAR CAPILLARY

CAPSULAR SPACE

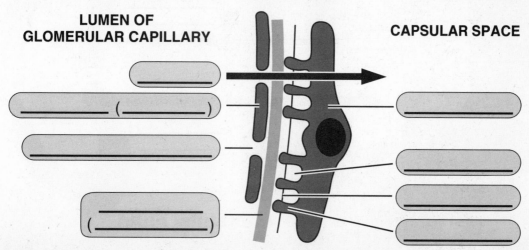

RENAL TUBULE HISTOLOGY :
Proximal Convoluted Tubule (PCT)

Cuboidal Epithelial Cells

The _____ border on the _____ surface (luminal surface) of the cells lining the
PCT increase the _____ available for the _____ of solutes and water.

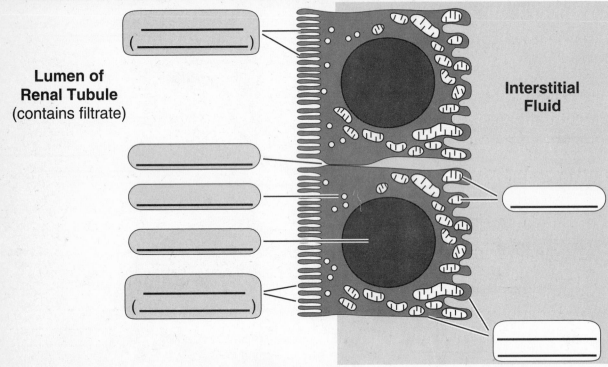

**Lumen of
Renal Tubule**
(contains filtrate)

**Interstitial
Fluid**

Cross Section of the PCT

Proximal Convoluted Tubule

Peritubular Capillary

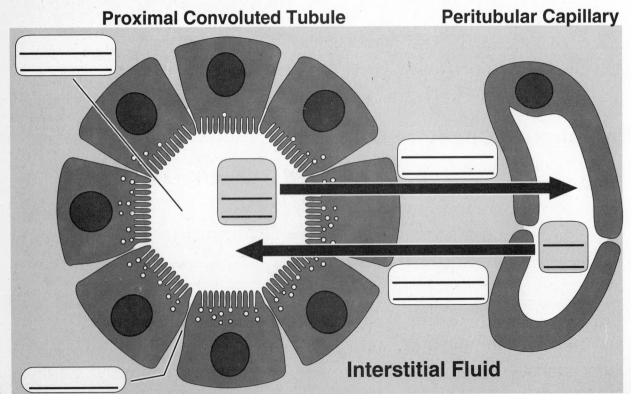

Interstitial Fluid

RENAL TUBULE HISTOLOGY :
Distal Convoluted Tubule (DCT) and Collecting Duct

Cuboidal Epithelial Cells

Most of the cells lining the DCT and collecting ducts are called _____.
Antidiuretic hormone (ADH) makes their apical membranes permeable to _____.
Principal cells are capable of secreting _____ ions.

Some of the cells lining the DCT and collecting ducts are called **Intercalated Cells**.
They are capable of secreting _____ ions.

Lumen of
Renal Tubule
(contains filtrate)

Interstitial
Fluid

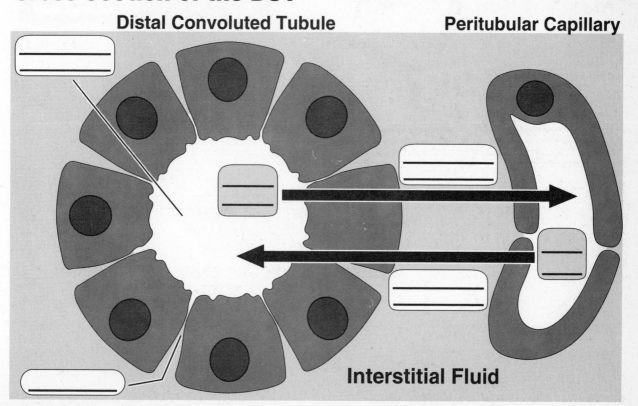

Cross Section of the DCT

Distal Convoluted Tubule

Peritubular Capillary

Interstitial Fluid

BLOOD SUPPLY TO KIDNEY

Only the arteries are shown in this illustration. The veins run parallel
to the arteries and have the same names.

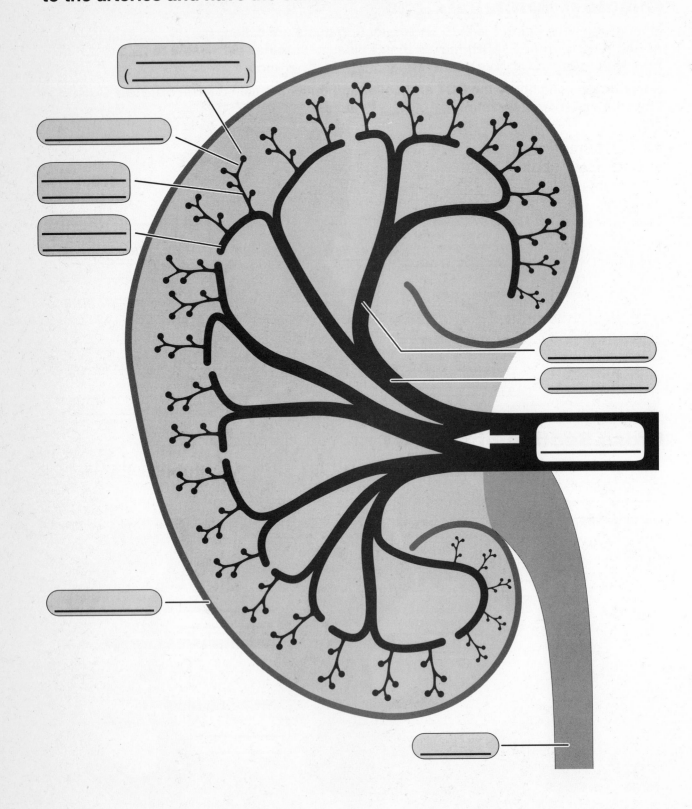

CORTICAL NEPHRON
Blood Supply

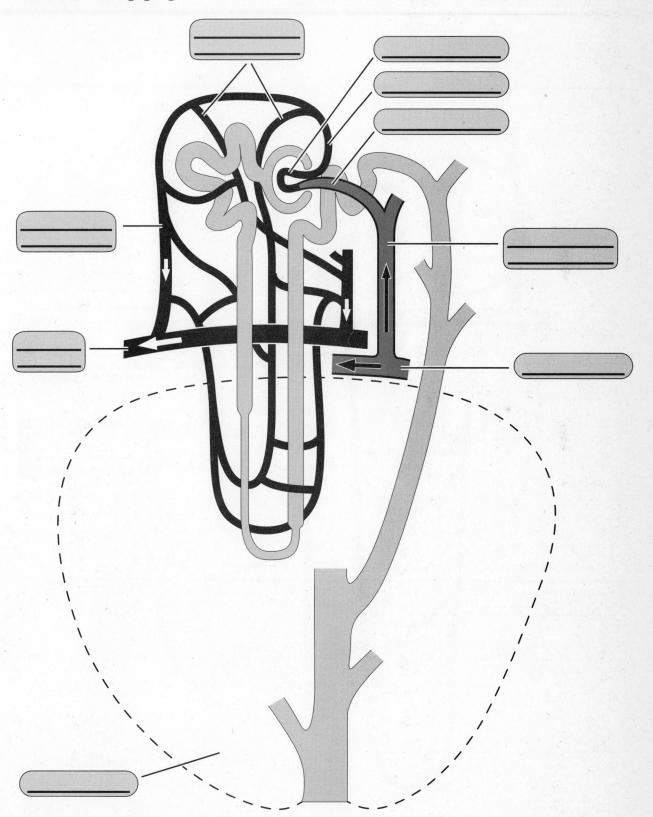

JUXTAMEDULLARY NEPHRON
Blood Supply

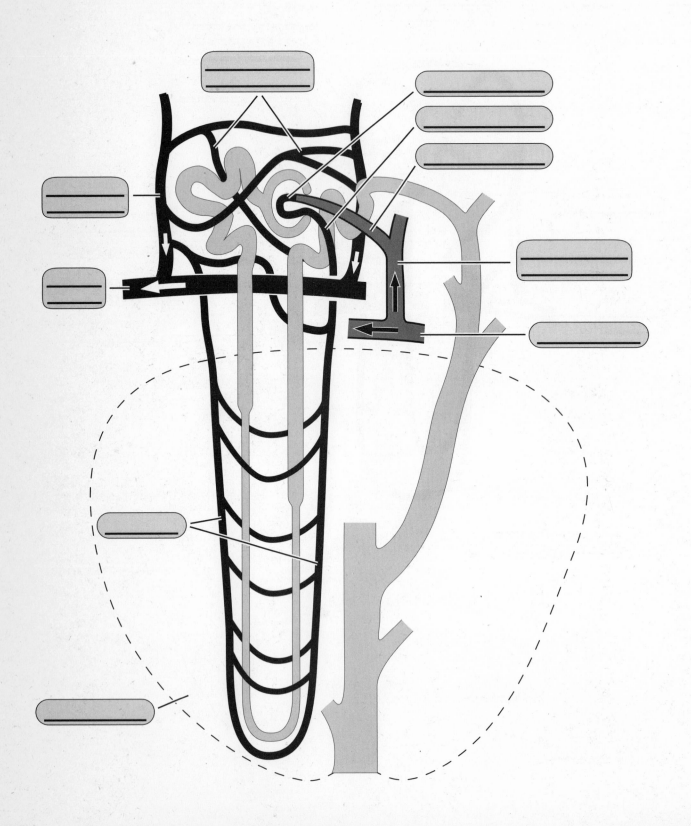

JUXTAGLOMERULAR APPARATUS

Juxtaglomerular Apparatus :
The juxtaglomerular apparatus is located next to (juxta) the _____ .
It has two parts, the _____ cells and the _____ .

Juxtaglomerular Cells :
Modified smooth muscle cells of the _____ arteriole.
They secrete the enzyme _____ .

Macula Densa :
Specialized cells of the _____ .
They are sensitive to _____ concentrations in the filtrate.

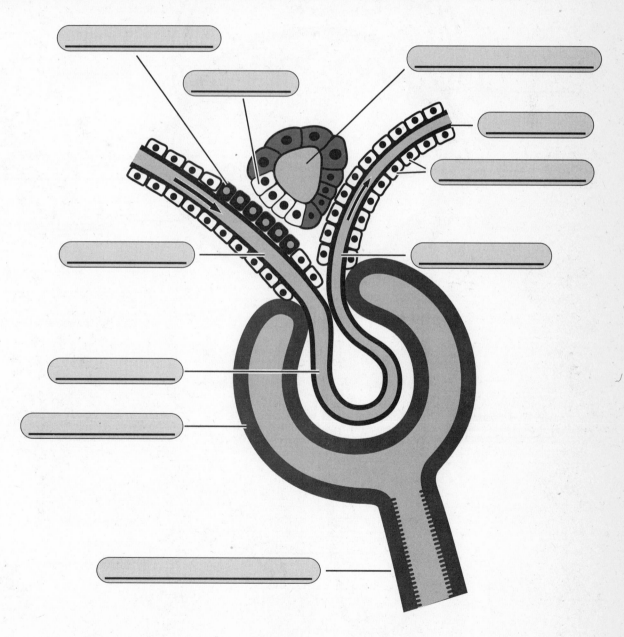

URINARY BLADDER AND URETHRA
Coronal Section (Female)

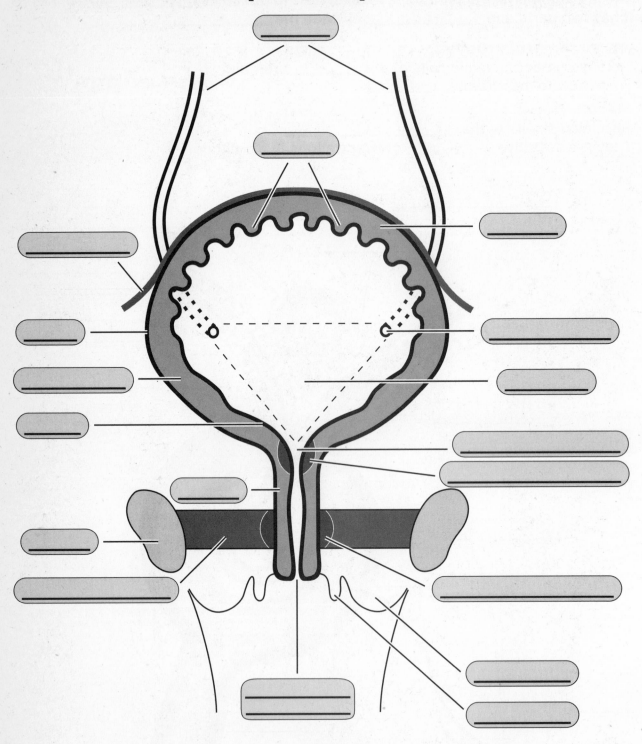

MICTURITION

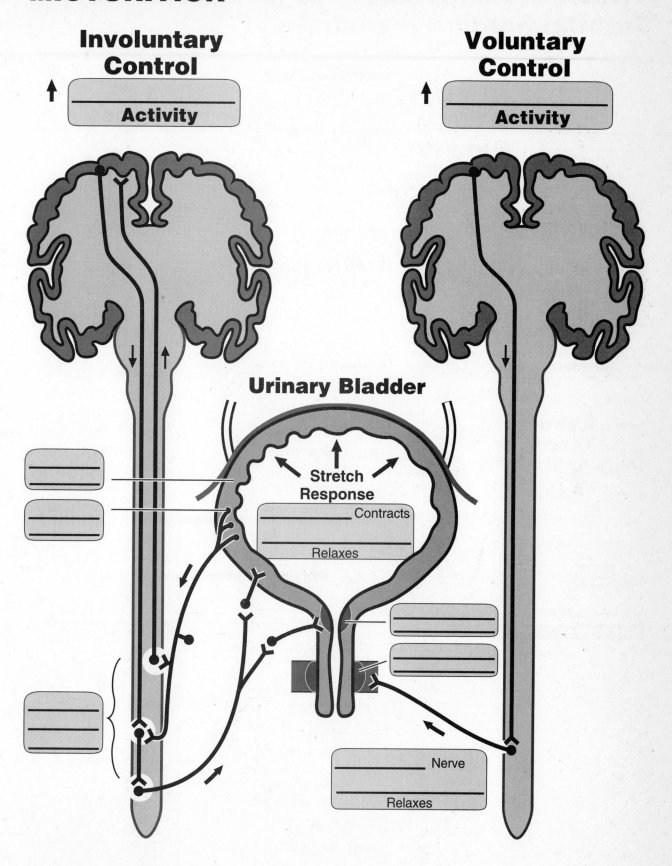

Involuntary Control

↑ _____
Activity

Voluntary Control

↑ _____
Activity

Urinary Bladder

Stretch Response

Contracts
_____
_____
Relaxes

_____ Nerve
_____
Relaxes

URINE FORMATION
Diagrammatic

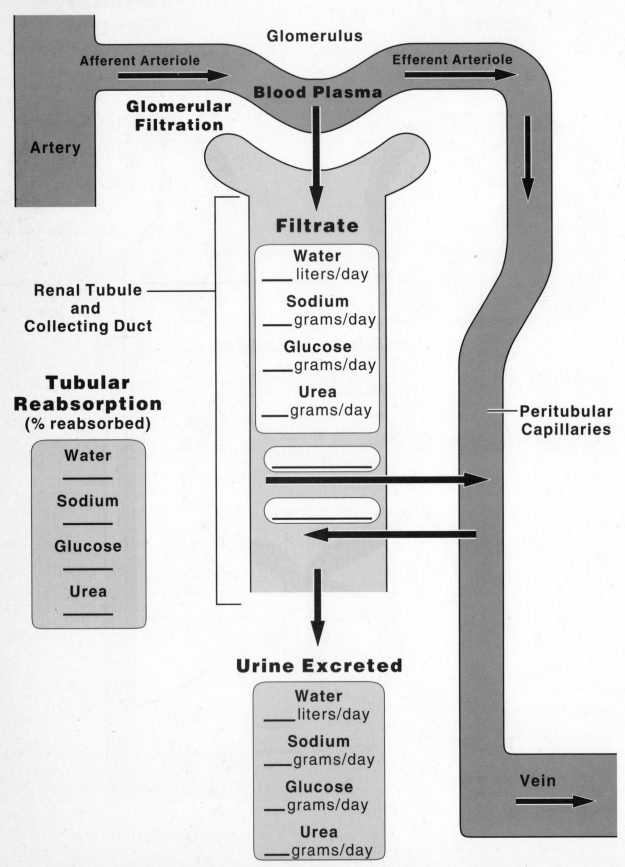

Glomerulus

Afferent Arteriole

Efferent Arteriole

Blood Plasma

Glomerular Filtration

Artery

Filtrate

Water
____ liters/day

Sodium
____ grams/day

Glucose
____ grams/day

Urea
____ grams/day

Renal Tubule
and
Collecting Duct

Peritubular Capillaries

Tubular Reabsorption
(% reabsorbed)

Water
____

Sodium
____

Glucose
____

Urea
____

Urine Excreted

Water
____ liters/day

Sodium
____ grams/day

Glucose
____ grams/day

Urea
____ grams/day

Vein

SODIUM PUMP (Na$^+$ / K$^+$ ATP–ase)

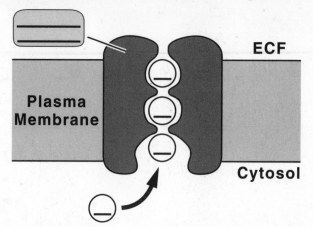

ECF

Plasma Membrane

Cytosol

Sodium in the cytosol binds to the _____ .

_____ concentration is low in the cytosol relative to the ____ .

_____ concentration is high in the cytosol relative to the ECF.

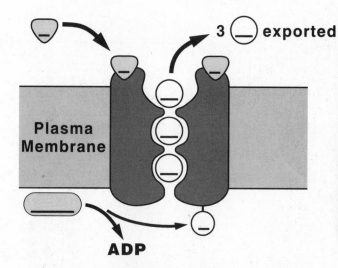

3 ⊖ exported

Plasma Membrane

ADP

_____ triggers the breakdown of ATP into ADP and the attachment of a high-energy phosphate group to the _____ .

This changes the shape of the pump protein so that the _____ ions are pushed through the membrane and _____ into the ECF.

Now the shape of the pump favors binding of ____ in the ECF.

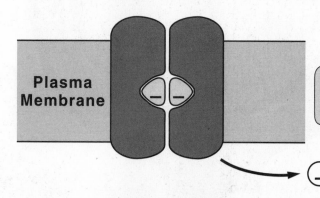

Plasma Membrane

K$^+$ binding triggers the release of _____ , again causing the shape of the _____ to change.

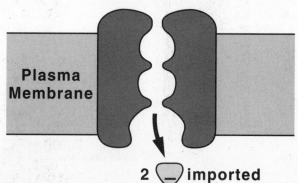

Plasma Membrane

K$^+$ is pushed through the membrane into the _____ , as the pump returns to its original shape.

The cycle repeats itself.

2 ⊖ imported

NET FILTRATION PRESSURE

NFP = GBHP – (CHP + BCOP)

NFP = _____ = 18 mm Hg

GBHP = _____ = 60 mm Hg

CHP = _____ = 15 mm Hg

BCOP = _____ = 27 mm Hg

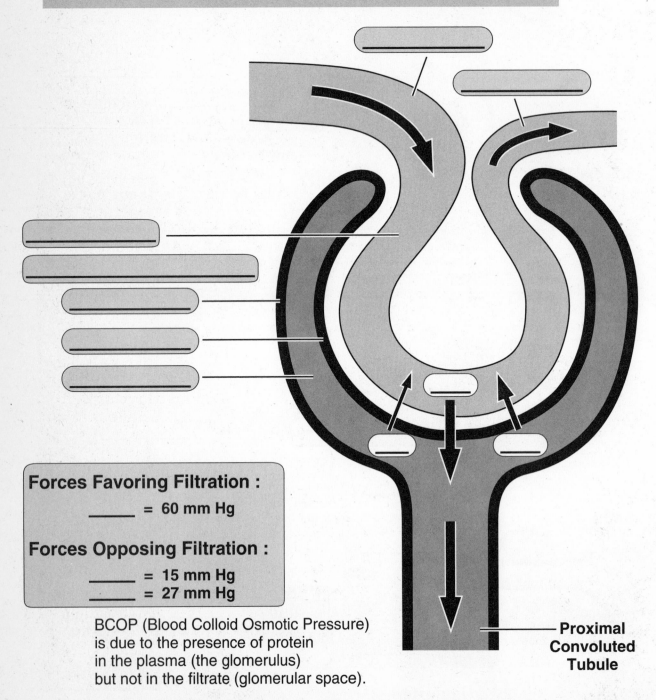

Forces Favoring Filtration :

_____ = 60 mm Hg

Forces Opposing Filtration :

_____ = 15 mm Hg

_____ = 27 mm Hg

BCOP (Blood Colloid Osmotic Pressure)
is due to the presence of protein
in the plasma (the glomerulus)
but not in the filtrate (glomerular space).

**Proximal
Convoluted
Tubule**

PROXIMAL CONVOLUTED TUBULE

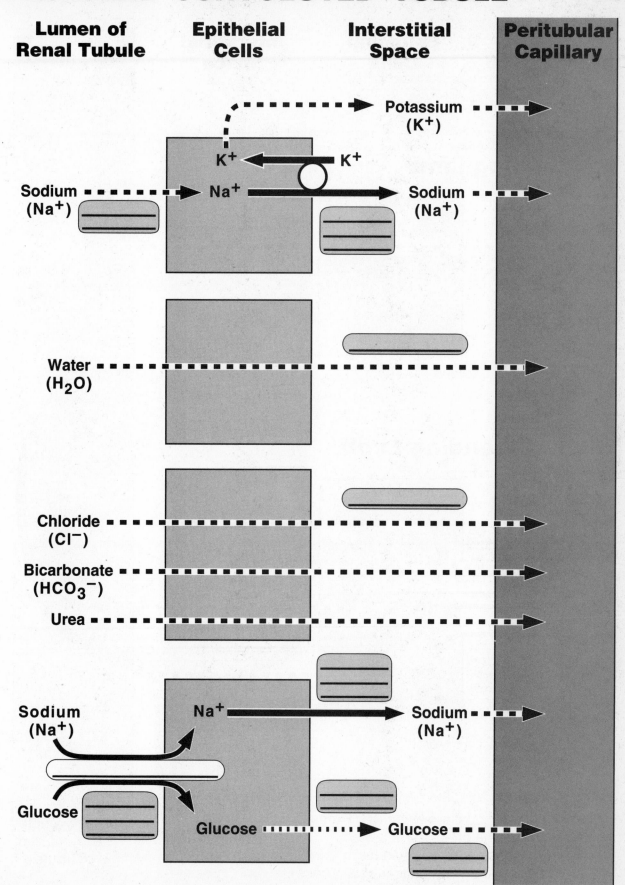

LOOP OF HENLE

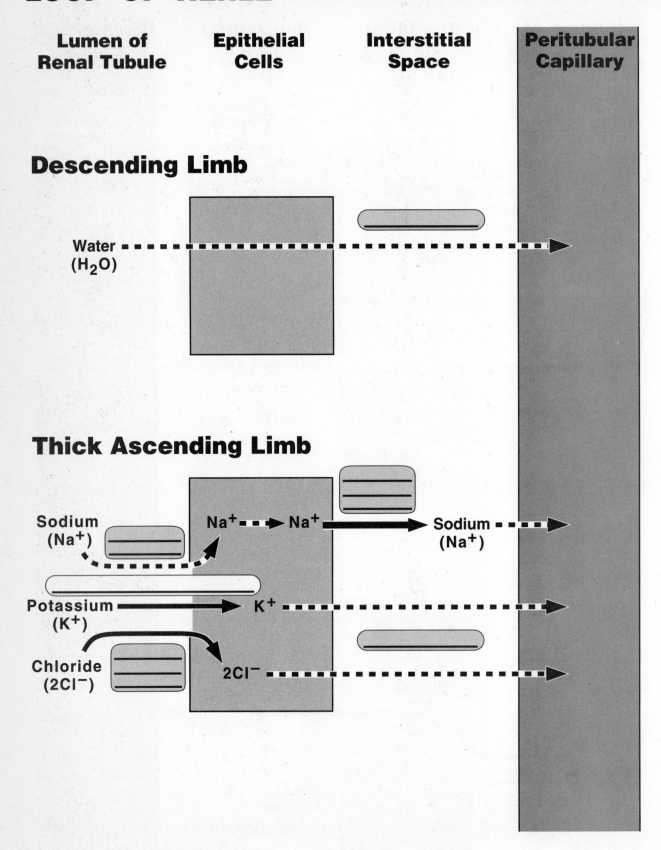

Lumen of Renal Tubule **Epithelial Cells** **Interstitial Space** **Peritubular Capillary**

Descending Limb

Water (H_2O)

Thick Ascending Limb

Sodium (Na^+)

Na^+ → Na^+ → Sodium (Na^+)

Potassium (K^+)

K^+

Chloride ($2Cl^-$)

$2Cl^-$

DCT AND COLLECTING DUCTS

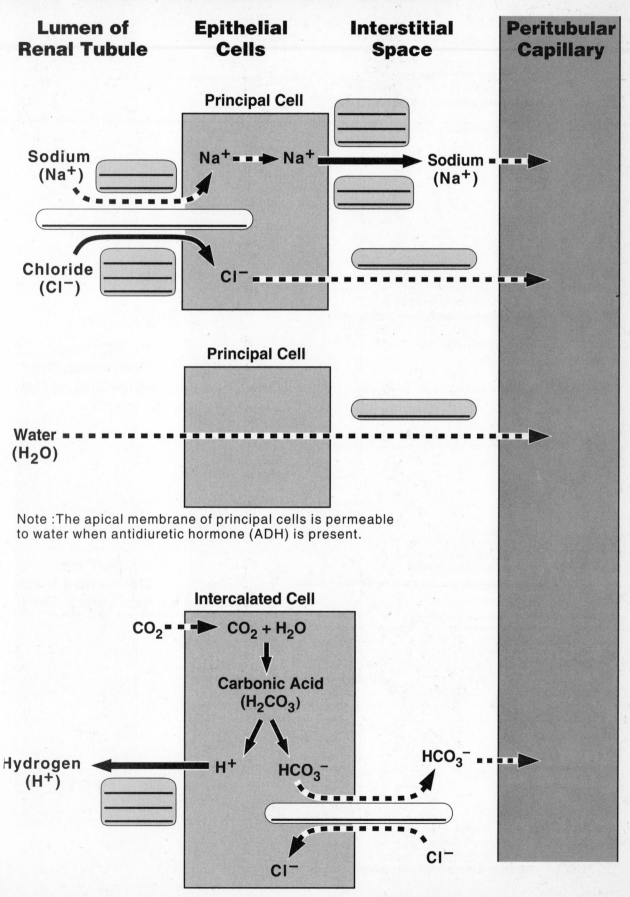

Note : The apical membrane of principal cells is permeable to water when antidiuretic hormone (ADH) is present.

TUBULAR SECRETION

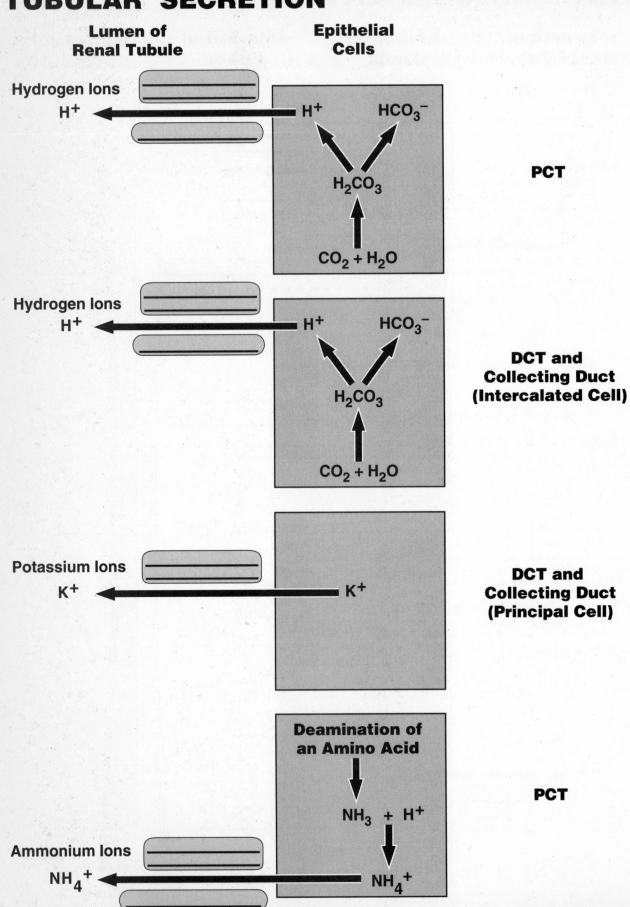

**Lumen of
Renal Tubule**

**Epithelial
Cells**

Hydrogen Ions
H^+

H^+ HCO_3^-

H_2CO_3

$CO_2 + H_2O$

PCT

Hydrogen Ions
H^+

H^+ HCO_3^-

H_2CO_3

$CO_2 + H_2O$

**DCT and
Collecting Duct
(Intercalated Cell)**

Potassium Ions
K^+

K^+

**DCT and
Collecting Duct
(Principal Cell)**

**Deamination of
an Amino Acid**

$NH_3 + H^+$

PCT

Ammonium Ions
NH_4^+

NH_4^+

FORMATION OF DILUTE URINE

Plasma ADH is _____ .

The heavy line represents the regions that are virtually impermeable to _____ in the absence of antidiuretic hormone (ADH).

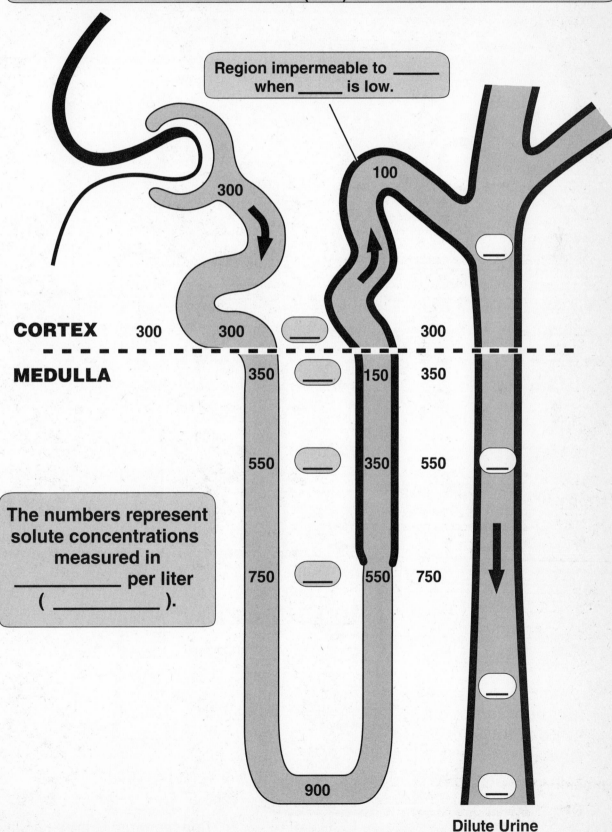

Region impermeable to _____ when _____ is low.

100

300

CORTEX   300   300   _____   300

MEDULLA   350   _____   150   350

              550   _____   350   550

The numbers represent solute concentrations measured in _____ per liter (_____).

              750   _____   550   750

              900

Dilute Urine

FORMATION OF CONCENTRATED URINE

Plasma ADH is _____ .

The heavy line in the thick ascending limb of the loop of Henle indicates the presence of _____ symporters.

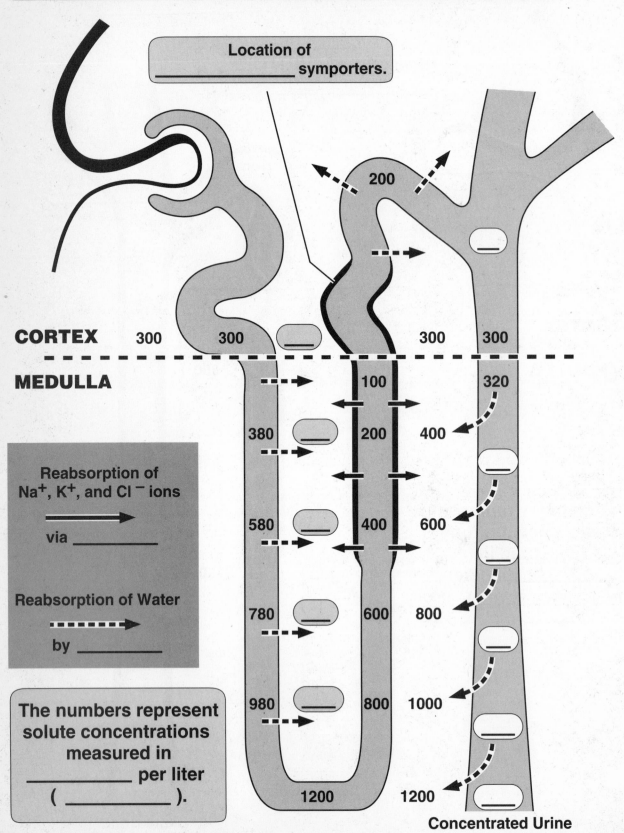

Location of _____ symporters.

CORTEX   300   300   [ ]   300   300

MEDULLA   380   200   100   320

Reabsorption of Na+, K+, and Cl⁻ ions

via _____

Reabsorption of Water

by _____

The numbers represent solute concentrations measured in _____ per liter (_____).

380   200   400

580   400   600

780   600   800

980   800   1000

1200   1200

Concentrated Urine

RECYCLING OF SALTS AND UREA

The _____ flow of blood in the vasa recta prevents washing away of the _____ that have accumulated in the _____ of the medulla.

As blood flows down the _____ portion of the vasa recta, NaCl and urea duffuse into the _____ from the surrounding _____ .

As blood flows up the _____ portion of the vasa recta, NaCl and urea diffuse from the _____ into the _____ .

Because of the arrangement of the ascending and descending portions of the vasa recta, _____ remain concentrated in the _____ .

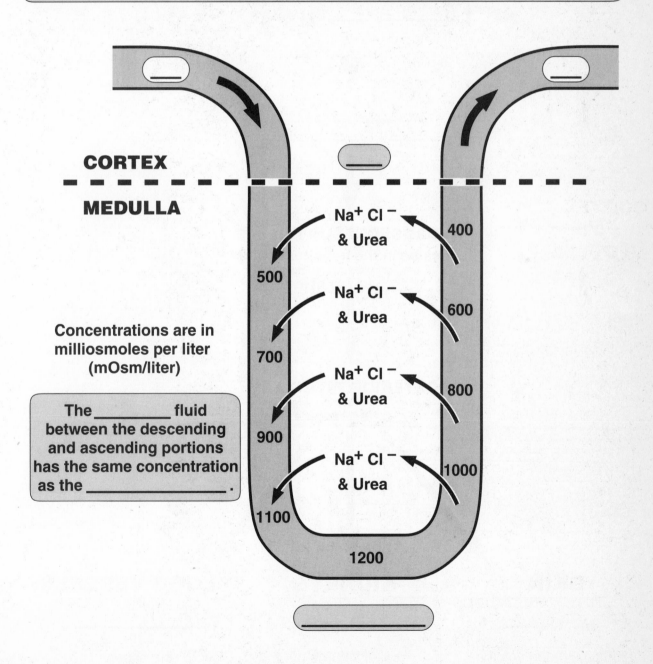

CORTEX

MEDULLA

Na⁺ Cl⁻ & Urea

400

500

Na⁺ Cl⁻ & Urea

600

700

Concentrations are in milliosmoles per liter (mOsm/liter)

Na⁺ Cl⁻ & Urea

800

900

The _____ fluid between the descending and ascending portions has the same concentration as the _____ .

Na⁺ Cl⁻ & Urea

1000

1100

1200

SECRETION OF ANTIDIURETIC HORMONE

Dehydration

Blood Water Concentration Below Normal

due to
_____
_____
_____

↑ _____ **Pressure**

(_____)
(_____)

NEUROSECRETORY CELLS
(located in the hypothalamus)

↑ _____ **production**

POSTERIOR PITUITARY

↑ _____ **secretion**

SKIN

↓ _____

maintains blood volume
and blood pressure

KIDNEYS

↑ _____

small volume of
concentrated urine
produced

BLOOD VESSELS

↑ _____

increases
blood pressure

URINE

Characteristics

Volume	**_____ liters (quarts) per day** (influenced by many factors)
Color	**_____ or _____** (varies with concentration and diet)
Turbidity	**_____ when fresh** (becomes cloudy)
Odor	**_____** (becomes ammonia-like)
pH	**Averages ____** (ranges between 4.6 and 8.0)
Specific Gravity	**____ – ____** (denser than water)

Organic Solutes

_____	**Urea; Creatinine; Uric Acid**
_____	**Derived from Benzoic Acid**
_____	**Derived from Indole**
_____	**Derived from Triglycerides**

Inorganic Solutes

Cations	_____ ; _____ ; _____ ; _____ ; _____
Anions	_____ ; _____ ; _____

95

FLUID COMPARTMENTS

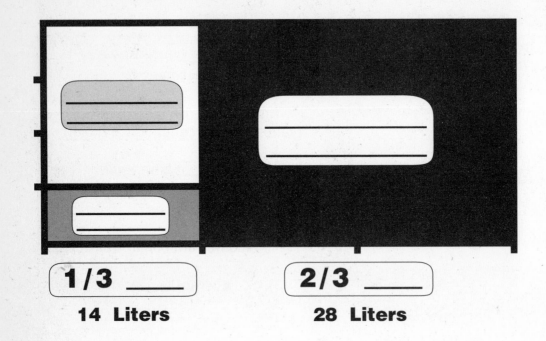

1/3 _____   2/3 _____

14 Liters   **28 Liters**

CAPILLARY BED

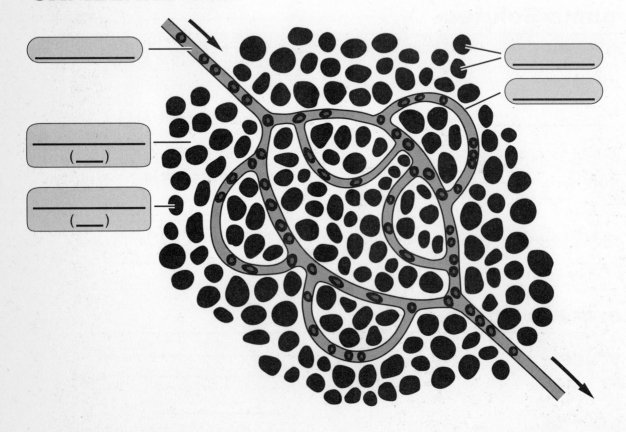

FLUID INTAKE AND OUTPUT

FLUID INTAKE
Total = _____ ml

_____
_____ ml

_____
_____ ml

_____
_____ ml

FLUID OUTPUT
Total = _____ ml

_____
_____ ml

_____
_____ ml

_____
_____ ml

_____
_____ ml

FACTORS THAT STIMULATE THIRST

Dehydration stimulates thirst in at least three ways :
(1) A decrease in _____ production leads to dryness of the mouth and pharynx.
(2) An increase in _____ pressure stimulates osmoreceptors.
(3) A decrease in _____ and _____ stimulates the release of renin.

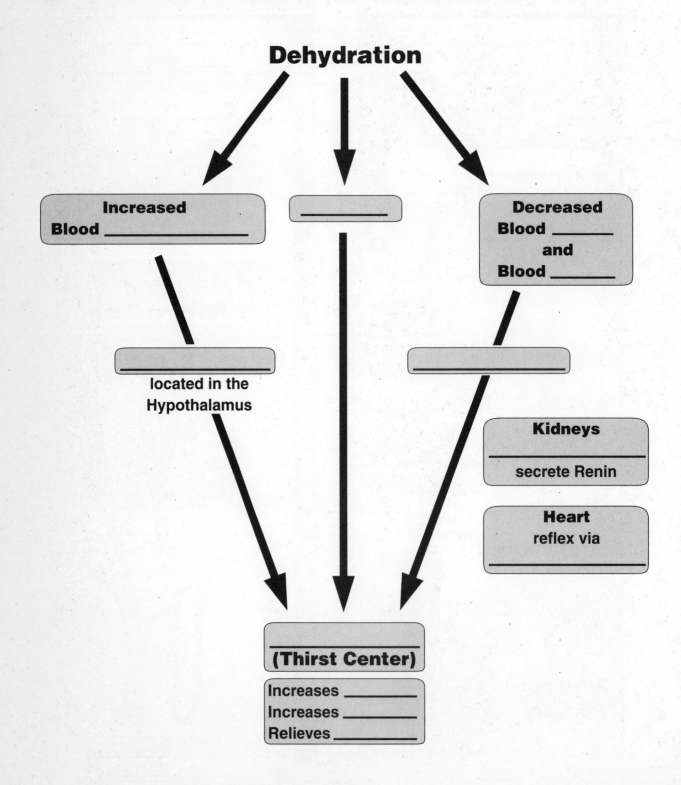

Dehydration

Increased
Blood _____

_____

Decreased
Blood _____
and
Blood _____

_____
located in the
Hypothalamus

_____

Kidneys
_____
secrete Renin

Heart
reflex via
_____

_____
(Thirst Center)

Increases _____
Increases _____
Relieves _____

ANTIDIURETIC HORMONE

Antidiuretic hormone (ADH) causes the _____ cells of the late DCT and _____ to be permeable to _____ .

Water loss or gain that is out of proportion to _____ loss or gain causes a change in the _____ of body fluids.

The receptors that monitor changes in the osmolarity of body fluids are called _____ and are located in the _____ .
They initiate the reflexes controlling _____ secretion.

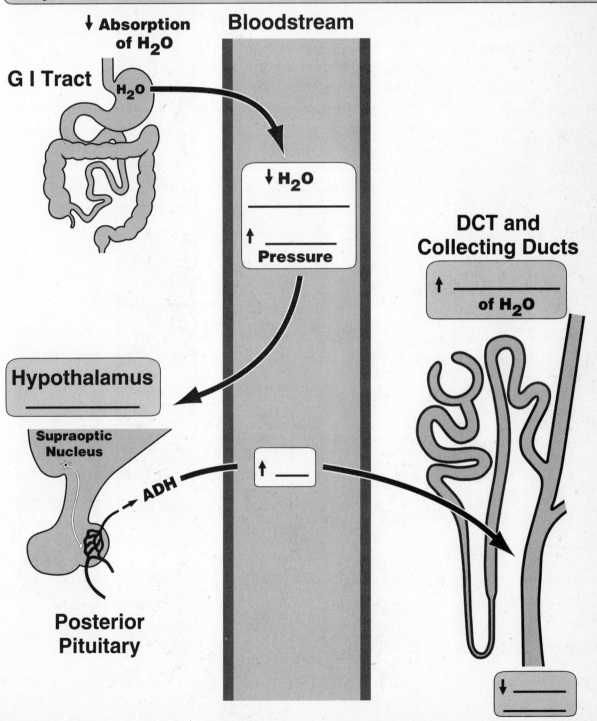

↓ Absorption of H$_2$O

Bloodstream

G I Tract

H$_2$O

↓ H$_2$O
_____
↑ _____
Pressure

DCT and Collecting Ducts

↑ _____
of H$_2$O

Hypothalamus
_____

Supraoptic Nucleus

ADH

↑ _____

Posterior Pituitary

↓ _____

ELECTROLYTE CONCENTRATIONS
Relative Concentrations of the Major Electrolytes (ions)

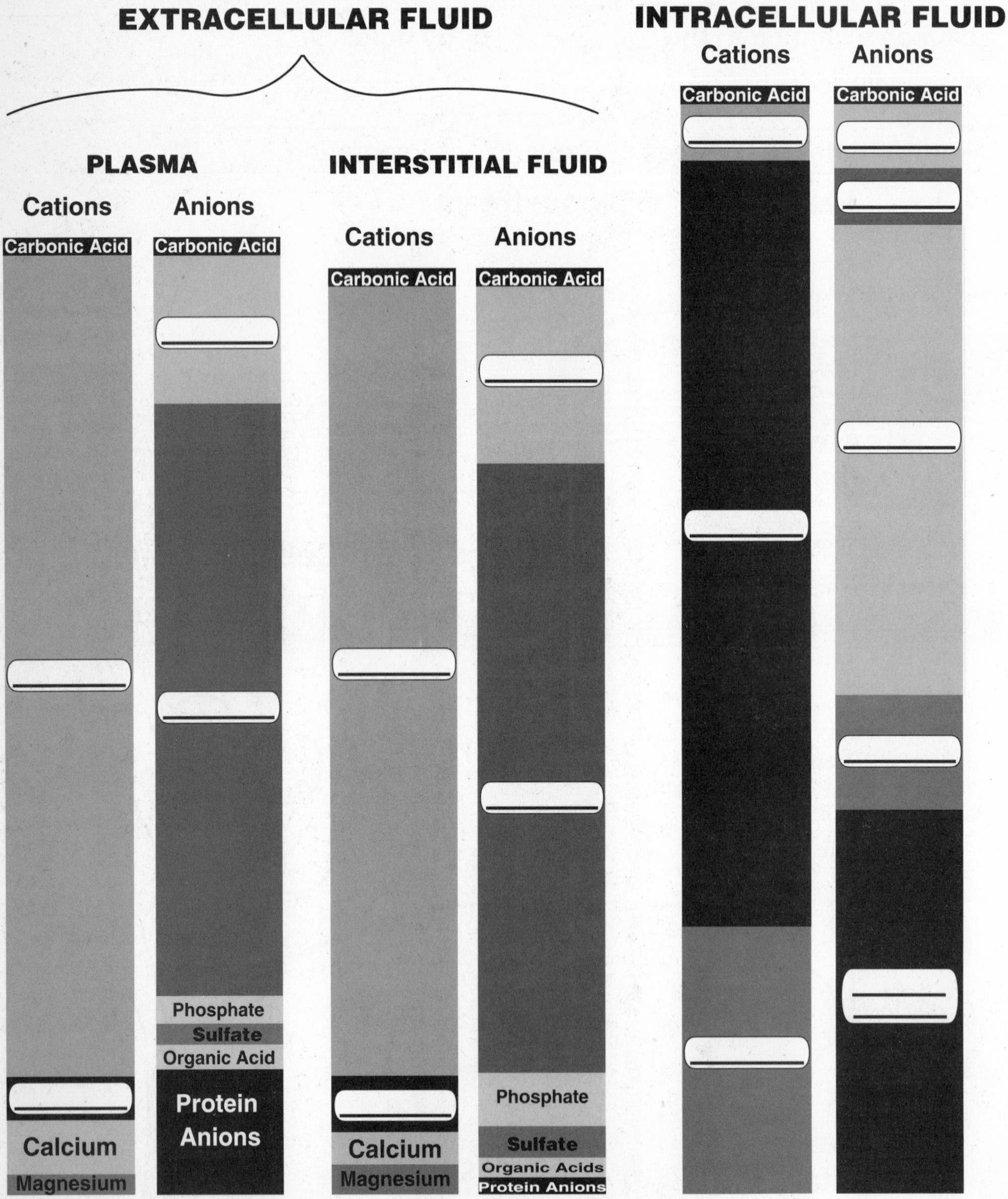

EXTRACELLULAR FLUID

INTRACELLULAR FLUID

Cations   Anions

Carbonic Acid   Carbonic Acid

PLASMA   **INTERSTITIAL FLUID**

Cations   Anions   Cations   Anions

Carbonic Acid   Carbonic Acid   Carbonic Acid   Carbonic Acid

Phosphate
Sulfate
Organic Acid

Protein
Anions

Phosphate

Sulfate

Calcium   Organic Acids
Magnesium   **Protein Anions**

Calcium
Magnesium

SODIUM BALANCE

Aldosterone _____ the plasma sodium (Na$^+$) concentration by increasing the rate of _____ in the DCT and collecting ducts.

Bloodstream

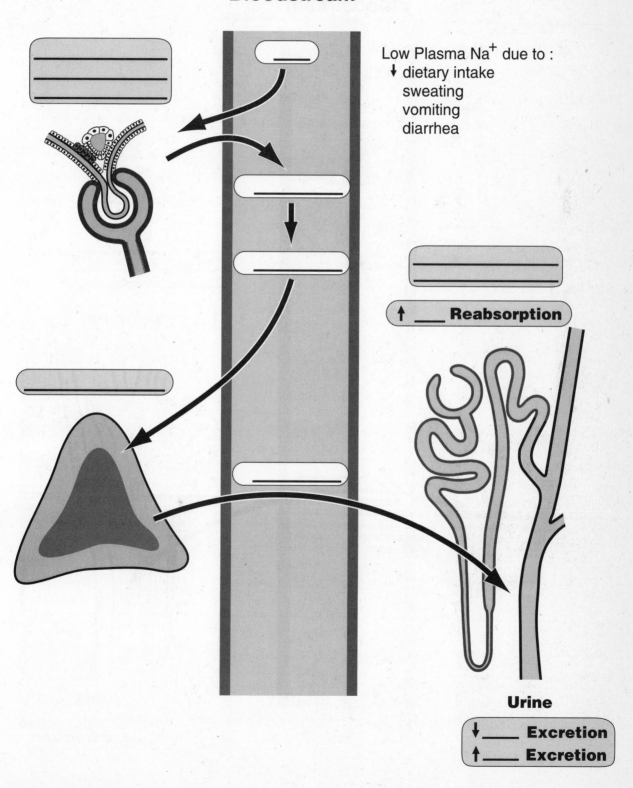

Low Plasma Na$^+$ due to :
- ↓ dietary intake
- sweating
- vomiting
- diarrhea

↑ ____ **Reabsorption**

Urine

↓ ____ **Excretion**
↑ ____ **Excretion**

POTASSIUM BALANCE

Aldosterone _____ the plasma potassium (K$^+$) concentration by increasing the rate of _____ in the DCT and collecting ducts.

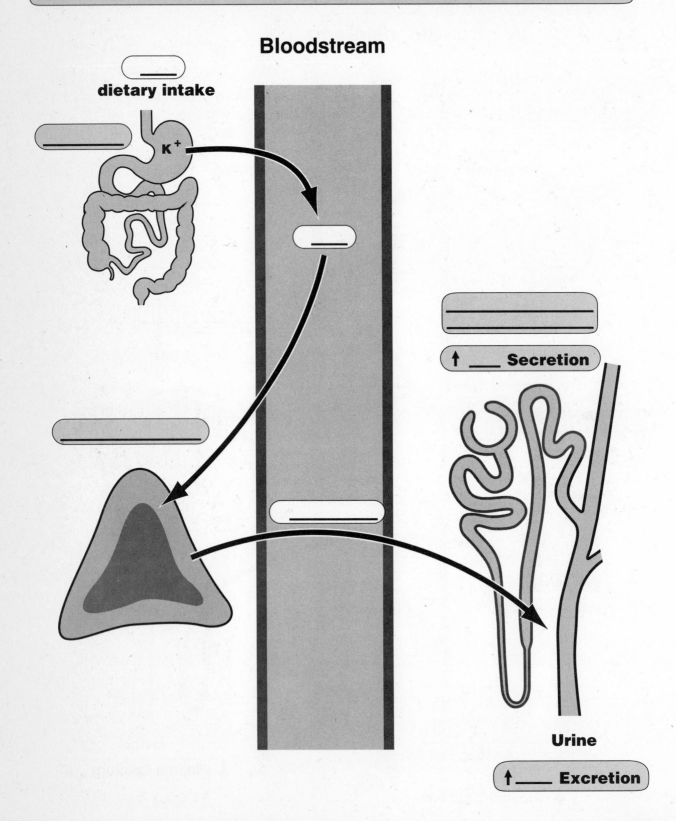

Bloodstream

dietary intake

K$^+$

↑ ____ **Secretion**

Urine

↑ ____ **Excretion**

CALCIUM BALANCE

Parathyroid hormone (PTH) _____ plasma calcium concentration by :
(1) stimulating the release of Ca^{2+} (calcium) from _____ ;
(2) stimulating the reabsorption of Ca^{2+} in _____ ;
(3) increasing the absorption of Ca^{2+} from the _____ .

Calcitonin (CT) _____ plasma calcium concentration by :
(1) stimulating the uptake of Ca^{2+} (calcium) by _____ ;
(2) increasing the excretion of Ca^{2+} in the _____ .

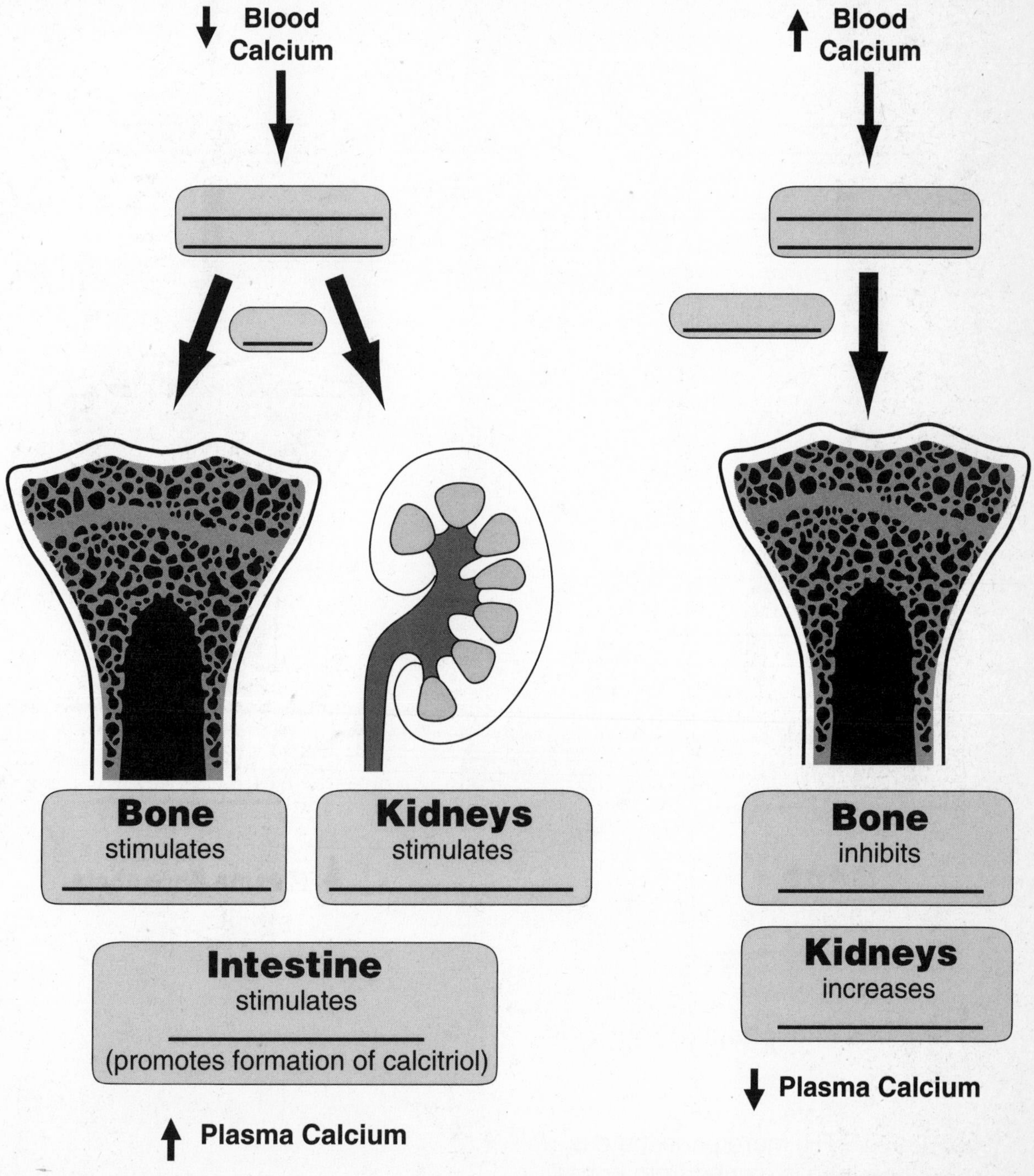

↓ Blood Calcium

↑ Blood Calcium

Bone
stimulates
_____

Kidneys
stimulates
_____

Bone
inhibits
_____

Intestine
stimulates
_____
(promotes formation of calcitriol)

Kidneys
increases
_____

↓ Plasma Calcium

↑ Plasma Calcium

PHOSPHATE BALANCE

PTH _____ plasma phosphate (HPO_4^{2-}) concentration by inhibiting the reabsorption of HPO_4^{2-} in _____ .

CT _____ plasma phosphate (HPO_4^{2-}) concentration by stimulating the uptake of HPO_4^{2-} by _____ .

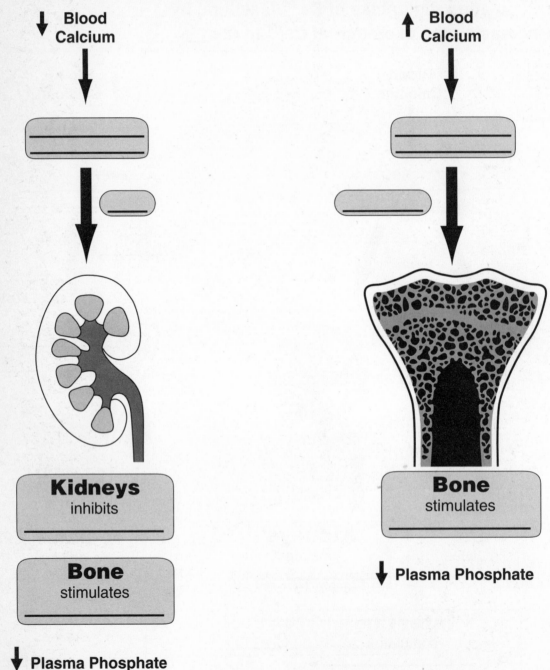

↓ Blood Calcium

↑ Blood Calcium

Kidneys
inhibits
_____

Bone
stimulates
_____

Bone
stimulates
_____

↓ Plasma Phosphate

↓ Plasma Phosphate

note :
in response to PTH, more phosphate is
lost in the urine than is gained from bones.

ELECTROLYTE IMBALANCE

Loss of Electrolytes

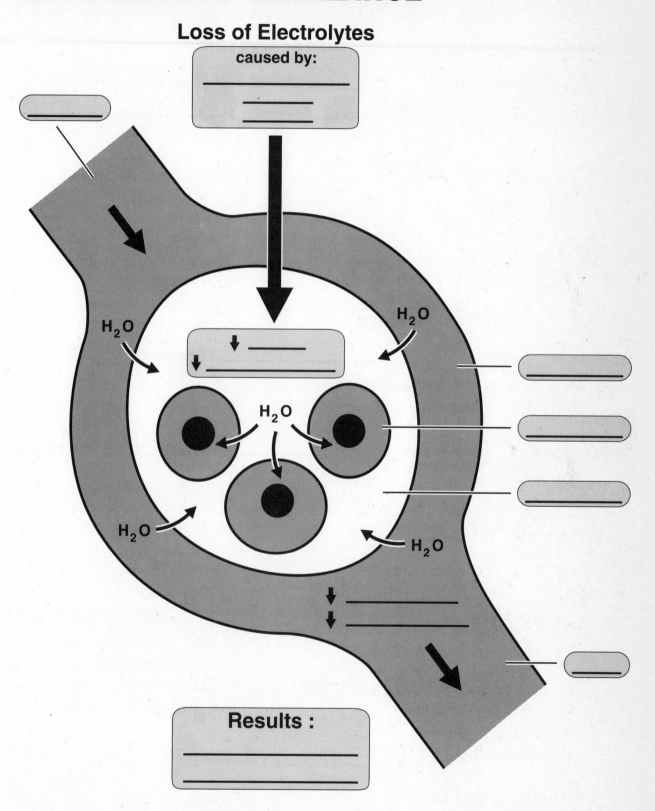

caused by:

Results :

BUFFER SYSTEMS

_____ **Buffer System**

Excess H$^+$ a weak base (_____) combines with H$^+$

$$HCO_3^- + \bigcirc \longrightarrow H_2CO_3 \longrightarrow H_2O + CO_2$$

Shortage of H$^+$ a weak acid (_____) dissociates, releasing H$^+$

$$H_2CO_3 \longrightarrow \bigcirc + HCO_3^-$$

_____ **Buffer System**

Excess H$^+$ a weak base (_____) combines with H$^+$

$$HPO_4^{2-} + \bigcirc \longrightarrow H_2PO_4^-$$

Shortage of H$^+$ a weak acid (_____) dissociates, releasing H$^+$

$$H_2PO_4^- \longrightarrow \bigcirc + HPO_4^{2-}$$

_____ **Buffer System**

Excess H$^+$ a weak base (_____) combines with H$^+$

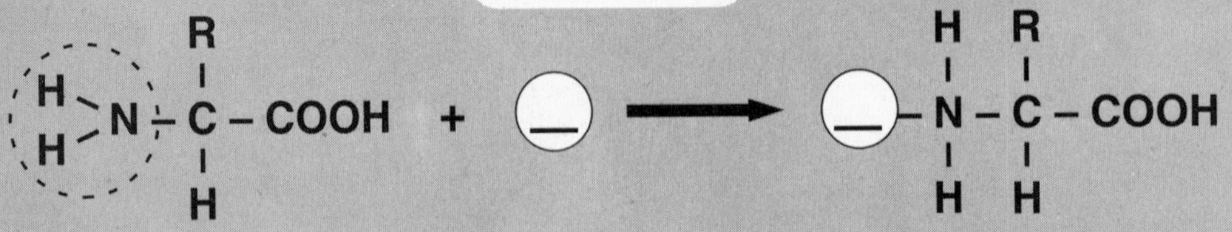

$$\overset{H}{\underset{H}{\,}}\!N\!-\!\overset{R}{\underset{H}{C}}\!-COOH + \bigcirc \longrightarrow \bigcirc\!-\!\overset{H}{\underset{H}{N}}\!-\!\overset{R}{\underset{H}{C}}\!-COOH$$

Shortage of H$^+$ a weak acid (_____) dissociates, releasing H$^+$

$$\overset{H}{\underset{H}{\,}}\!N\!-\!\overset{R}{\underset{H}{C}}\!-COOH \longrightarrow \bigcirc + \overset{H}{\underset{H}{\,}}\!N\!-\!\overset{R}{\underset{H}{C}}\!-COO^-$$

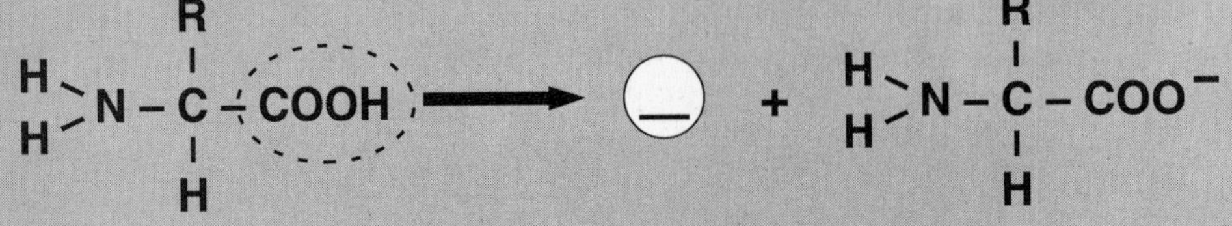

EXHALATION OF CARBON DIOXIDE

The pH of body fluids may be adjusted by a change in the rate and depth of breathing.

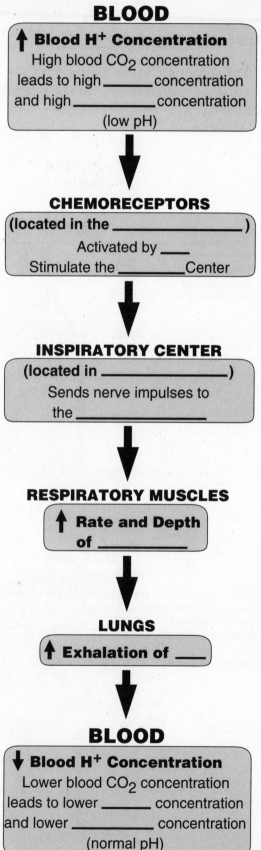

BLOOD

↑ **Blood H⁺ Concentration**

High blood CO_2 concentration leads to high _____ concentration and high _____ concentration

(low pH)

CHEMORECEPTORS

(located in the _____)

Activated by ____

Stimulate the _____ Center

INSPIRATORY CENTER

(located in _____)

Sends nerve impulses to the _____

RESPIRATORY MUSCLES

↑ **Rate and Depth**
of _____

LUNGS

↑ **Exhalation of ____**

BLOOD

↓ **Blood H⁺ Concentration**

Lower blood CO_2 concentration leads to lower _____ concentration and lower _____ concentration

(normal pH)

EXCRETION OF HYDROGEN IONS

Renal tubules may raise blood pH in three ways :
(1) Secretion (and excretion) of ___ .
(2) Reabsorption of filtered _____ .
(3) Synthesis and absorption of newly formed _____ .

In the PCT, H^+ ions are secreted by secondary active transport; HCO_3^- is reabsorbed by diffusion. Although the reabsorbed HCO_3^- and the filtered HCO_3^- are of different origins, filtered HCO_3^- disappears at the same time that the HCO_3^- formed in the cell enters the blood; so the net effect is the reabsorption of the filtered bicarbonate.

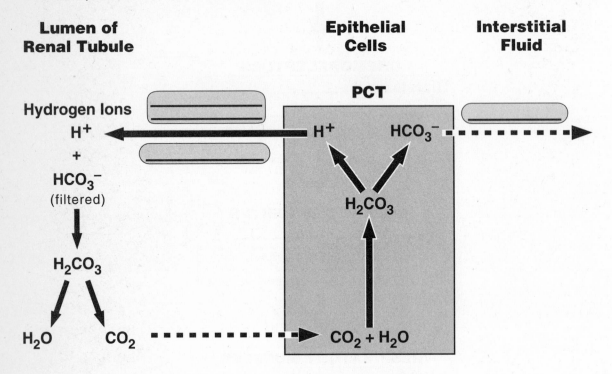

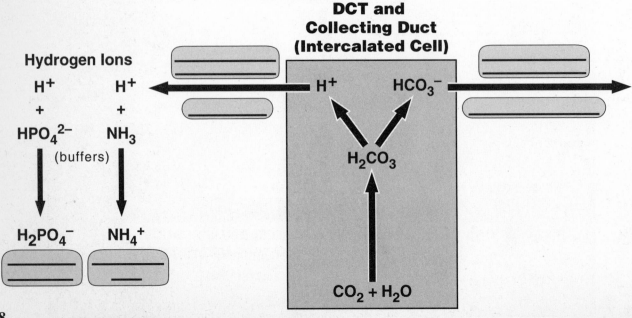

ACIDOSIS AND ALKALOSIS

Acidosis (pH below _____)

Respiratory Acidosis

Definition : pCO_2 above ___ mm Hg

Cause : _____

Compensation : increased excretion of ___
increased reabsorption of _____

Metabolic Acidosis

Definition : HCO_3^- below ___ mEq/liter

Cause : loss of _____ (diarrhea; ketosis; renal dysfunction)

Compensation : _____

Alkalosis (pH above _____)

Respiratory Alkalosis

Definition : pCO_2 below ___ mm Hg

Cause : _____

Compensation : decreased excretion of ___
decreased reabsorption of _____

Metabolic Alkalosis

Definition : HCO_3^- above ___ mEq/liter

Cause : loss of ____ (vomiting; diuretics; alkaline drugs)

Compensation : _____

Part III : Terminology

Pronunciation Guide

Pronunciation Key

Accented Syllables

The strongest accented syllable is in capital letters : dī - ag - NŌ - sis

Secondary accents are indicated by a prime (′) : fiz′ - ē - OL - ō - jē

Vowels

Long vowels are indicated by a horizontal line (macron) above the letter :

ā as in make   ē as in be   ī as in ivy   ō as in pole

Short vowels are unmarked :

e as in pet   i as in pit   o as in pot   u as in bud

Other Phonetic Symbols

a as in about   oo as in do   yoo as in cute   oy as in noise

---

acetone   AS - e - tōn
acetonuria   as′ - e - tō - NOO - rē - a
acidemia   as′ - i - DĒ - mē - a
acidosis   as′ - i - DŌ - sis
adenosine   a - DEN - ō - sēn
adipose   AD - i - pōs
adrenal   a - DRĒ - nal
afferent   AF - er - ent
albumin   al - BYOO - min
albuminuria   al′ - byoo - mi - NOO - rē - a
aldosterone   al - DA - ster - ōn
alkalemia   al′ - ka - LĒ - mē - a
alkalosis   al′ - ka - LŌ - sis
amine   a - MĒN
amino   a - MĒ - nō
angiotensin   an′ - jē - ō - TEN - sin
angiotensinogen   an′ - jē - ō - ten - SIN - ō - jen
anhydrase   an - HĪ - drās
anion   AN - ī - on
antidiuretic   an′ - ti - dī′ - yoo - RET - ik
antiport   AN - ti - port
anuria   a - NOO - rē - a
apical   AP - i - cal
arcuate   AR - kyoo - āt
areolar   a - RĒ - ō - lar
arteriole   ar - TĒ - rē - ōl
atrial   Ā - trē - al
autoregulation   aw′ - tō - reg′ - yoo - LĀ - shun

basolateral   bā′ - sō - LAT - er - al
benzoic   ben - ZŌ - ik
bicarbonate   bī - KAR - bō - nāt
bile   BĪL

bilirubin   bil′ - ē - ROO - bin
bilirubinuria   bil′ - ē - roo - bi - NOO - rē - a
biliverdin   bil′ - ē - VER - din
Bowman's   BŌ - manz

calcitonin   kal′ - si - TŌ - nin
calcitriol   kal - si - TRĪ - ol
calcium   KAL - sē - um
calculi   KAL - kyoo - lī
calculus   KAL - kyoo - lus
calyses   KĀ - li - sēz
calyx   KĀ - liks
candida albicans   KAN - di - da AL - bi - kanz
capillary   KAP - i - lar′ - ē
capsular   KAP - soo - lar
carbonic   kar - BON - ik
carboxyl   kar - BOK - sil
catheter   KATH - i - ter
catheterization   kath′ - i - ter - i - ZĀ - shun
cation   KAT - ī - on
chloride   KLOR - īd
columnar   kol - LUM - nar
colloid   KOL - oyd
convoluted   KON - vō - loo - ted
coronal   kō - RŌ - nal
corpuscle   KOR - pus - sul
creatinine   krē - AT - i - nin
cuboidal   kyoo - BOY - dal

deamination   dē - am′ - i - NĀ - shun
deciliter   DES - i - lē′ - ter
detrusor   de - TROO - ser
diabetes insipidus   dī - a - BĒ - tēz in - SIP - i - dus

112

diabetes mellitus dī-a-BĒ-tēz MEL-i-tus
dialysate dī-AL-i-sāt
dialysis dī-AL-i-sis
diffusion dif-YOO-zhun
dihydrogen dī-HĪ-drō-jen
distal DIS-tal
diuresis dī′-yoo-RĒ-sis
diuretic dī′-yoo-RET-ik

efferent EF-er-ent
electrolyte e-LEK-trō-līt
endocytosis en′-dō-sī-TŌ-sis
endothelial en′-dō-THĒ-lē-al
endothelium en′-dō-THĒ-lē-um
epithelial ep′-i-THĒ-lē-al
epithelium ep′-i-THĒ-lē-um
enuresis en′-yoo-RĒ-sis
enzyme EN-zīm
erythropoiesis e-rith′-rō-poy-Ē-sis
erythropoietin e-rith′-rō-POY-ē-tin
excretion eks-KRĒ-shun
exocytosis eks′-ō-sī-TŌ-sis

fascia FASH-ē-a
feces FĒ-sēz
fenestration fen′-es-TRĀ-shun
filtrate FIL-trāt

glomerular glō-MER-yoo-lar
glomeruli glō-MER-yoo-lī
glomerulus glō-MER-yoo-lus
gluconeogenesis gloo′-kō-nē′-ō-JEN-e-sis
glucose GLOO-kōs
glucosuria gloo′-kō-SOO-rē-a
glycosuria glī′-kō-SOO-rē-a

hematuria hē′-ma-TOOR-ē-a
hemodialysis hē′-mō-dī-AL-i-sis
Henle HEN-lē
hilum HĪ-lum
hilus HĪ-lus
hippuric hip-YOOR-ik
homeostasis hō′-mē-ō-STĀ-sis
hydrochloric hī′-drō-KLOR-ik
hydrogen HĪ-drō-jen
hydrostatic hī′-drō-STAT-ik
hydroxide hī-DROK-sīd
hydroxyl hī-DROK-sil
hypercalcemia hī′-per-kal-SĒ-mē-a
hyperkalemia hī′-per-ka-LĒ-mē-a
hypermagnesemia hī′-per-mag′-ne-SĒ-mē-a
hypernatremia hī′-per-na-TRĒ-mē-a
hyperosmotic hī′-per-os-MOT-ik
hyperphosphatemia hī′-per-fos′-fa-TĒ-mē-a

hypertonic hī′-per-TON-ik
hypocalcemia hī′-pō-kal-SĒ-mē-a
hypochloremia hī′-pō-klō-RĒ-mē-a
hypokalemia hī′-pō-ka-LĒ-mē-a
hypomagnesemia hī′-pō-mag′-ne-SĒ-mē-a
hyponatremia hī′-pō-na-TRĒ-mē-a
hypo–osmotic hī′-pō-os-MOT-ik
hypophosphatemia hī′-pō-fos′-fa-TĒ-mē-a
hypotonic hī′-pō-TON-ik
hypovolemia hī′-pō-vō-LĒ-mē-a

incontinence in-KON-ti-nens
indican IN-di-kan
indole IN-dōl
intercalated in-TER-ka-lāt-ed
interlobar in′-ter-LŌ-bar
interlobular in′-ter-LOB-yoo-lar
interstitial in′-ter-STISH-al
interstitium in′-ter-STISH-i-um
inulin IN-yoo-lin
ion Ī-on
iso–osmotic ī′-sō-oz-MOT-ik
isosmotic ī-sos-MOT-ik
isotonic ī-sō-TON-ik

juxta JUKS-ta
juxtaglomerular juks′-ta-glō-MER-yoo-lar
juxtamedullary juks′-ta-MED-yoo-lar′-ē

ketone KĒ-tōn
ketosis kē-TŌ-sis

lamina propria LAM-i-na PRŌ-prē-a
lithotripsy LITH-ō-trip′-sē
Littre LĒ-tra
lumen LOO-men
luminal LOO-mi-nal

macula densa MAK-yoo-la DEN-sa
magnesium mag-NĒ-zē-um
medulla me-DULL-a
medullary MED-yoo-lar′-ē
membranous MEM-bra-nus
metabolic met′-a-BOL-ik
metabolism me-TAB-ō-lizm
metabolite me-TAB-ō-līt
microvilli mī-krō-VIL-ī
microvillus mī-krō-VIL-us
micturition mik′-too-RISH-un
milliequivalent mil′-ē-ē-KWIV-a-lent
millimole MIL-ē-mōl
milliosmole mil′-ē-OZ-mōl
monohydrogen mon-ō-HĪ-drō-jen
mucosa myoo-KŌ-sa

113

mucosae myoo-KŌ-sē
mucous MYOO-kus
mucus MYOO-kus
muscularis mus-kyoo-LAR-is

nanometer NAN-a-mē-ter
natriuretic na′-trē-yoo-RET-ik
nephrology ne-FROL-ō-jē
nephron NEF-ron
nonelectrolyte non′-e-LEK-trō-līt

orifice OR-i-fis
osmolarity oz′-mō-LAR-i-tē
osmoreceptor oz′-mō-re-SEP-tor
osmosis os-MŌ-sis
osmotic oz-MOT-ik

papilla pa-PIL-a
papillae pa-PIL-ē
papillary PAP-i-lar′-ē
para–aminohippuric par′-a-a-MĒ-nō-hip-YOOR-ik
parenchyma pa-REN-ki-ma
parietal pa-RĪ-e-tal
pedicel PED-i-sul
penis PĒ-nis
peptide PEP-tīd
peristalsis per′-i-STAL-sis
peristaltic per′-i-STAL-tik
peritoneal per′-i-tō-NĒ-al
peritoneum per′-i-tō-NĒ-um
peritubular per′-i-TOO-byoo-lar
phagocytosis fag′-ō-sī-TŌ-sis
phosphate FOS-fāt
phosphorus FOS-for-us
pinocytosis pi′-nō-sī-TŌ-sis
plexus PLEK-sus
podocyte POD-ō-sīt
potassium pō-TAS-ē-um
prostate PROS-tāt
prostatic pros-TAT-ik
proximal PROK-si-mal
pyria pī-YOO-rē-a

renal RĒ-nal
renin RĒ-nin
respiratory RES-per-a-tor′-ē
retroperitoneal re′-trō-per-i-tō-NĒ-al
ruga ROO-ga
rugae ROO-jē

saline SĀ-lēn
serosa sēr-Ō-sa
serous SĒR-us
sodium SŌ-dē-um

solute SOL-yoot
sphincter SFINGK-ter
squamous SKWĀ-mus
Starling's STAR-lingz
submucosa sub-myoo-KŌ-sa
substrate SUB-strāt
sudoriferous soo′-dor-IF-er-us
sulfate SUL-fāt
suprarenal soo′-pra-RĒ-nal
symport SIM-port

trichomonas trik′-ō-MŌ-nas
trigone TRĪ-gōn
tubule TOO-byool
turbidity tur-BID-i-tē

urea yoo-RĒ-a
uremia yoo-RĒ-mē-a
ureter yoo-RĒ-tur
ureteral yoo-RĒ-tur-al
ureteric yoo′-re-TER-ik
urethra yoo-RĒ-thra
urethral yoo-RĒ-thral
uric YOOR-ik
urinalysis yoor′-i-NAL-i-sis
urinary YOOR-i-nar′-ē
urinate YOOR-i-nāt
urination yoor-i-NĀ-shun
urine YOOR-in
urobilinogen yoo′-rō-bī-LIN-ō-jen
urobilinogenuria yoo-rō-bī-lin-ō-je-NOOR-ē-a
urogenital yoo′-rō-JEN-i-tal
urology yoo-ROL-ō-jē

vagina va-JĪ-na
vasa recta VĀ-sa REK-ta
vasoconstriction vas-ō-kon-STRIK-shun
vestibule VES-ti-byool
viscera VIS-er-a
visceral VIS-er-al

Glossary of Terms

Absorption   The passage of digested foods from the gastrointestinal tract into blood or lymph.

ACE   *See* Angiotensin converting enzyme.

Acetonuria   *See* Ketosis.

Acid   A proton donor, or substance that dissociates into hydrogen ions (H^+) and anions. It is characterized by an excess of hydrogen ions and a pH less than 7.

Acidemia   *See* Acidosis.

Acidic solution   A solution that contains more hydrogen ions (H^+) than hydroxyl ions (OH^-). A pH less than 7.

Acidosis   A condition in which blood pH is below 7.35. Also called *acidemia*.

Active processes   Energy-consuming processes that are used to move substances across plasma membranes. There are two basic types: active transport and bulk transport; both require energy derived from splitting ATP. These processes are used to move substances that cannot be moved by passive processes (the substances are too big, have the wrong charge, or must move against their concentration gradient).

Active transport   A mechanism for moving substances across plasma membranes that requires the energy derived from splitting ATP. Particular integral membrane proteins act as ATP-driven pumps to push certain ions and some smaller molecules across the plasma membrane. Ions actively transported include sodium, potassium, hydrogen, calcium, iodide, and chloride; small molecules actively transported include amino acids and monosaccharides. *Also see* Primary active transport and Secondary active transport.

Adenosine triphosphate (ATP)   The energy "currency" of all living cells; energy readily available for cellular activities. It is synthesized in a process called cellular respiration.

ADH   *See* Antidiuretic hormone.

Adipose capsule   The middle layer of tissue surrounding each kidney. It consists of fat cells (adipocytes).

Afferent   Carrying toward. Applies to blood vessels and nerves.

Afferent arteriole   In the kidney, a blood vessel that carries blood toward a glomerulus. It branches from an interlobular artery.

Albumin   The most abundant (60%) and smallest of the plasma proteins. It helps regulate the osmotic pressure of blood plasma.

Albuminuria   The presence of albumin in the urine.

Alcohol   A substance that acts as a diuretic (increases urine production) by inhibiting the secretion of antidiuretic hormone (ADH) by the posterior pituitary gland.

Aldosterone   A hormone secreted by the adrenal cortex. In the kidney, it increases the reabsorption of sodium by the principal cells of the collecting ducts; water follows sodium by osmosis, increasing blood volume and blood pressure. It stimulates the tubular secretion of potassium, so more potassium is excreted.

Alimentary canal   *See* Gastrointestinal tract.

Alkalemia   *See* Alkalosis.

Alkaline solution   A solution that contains more hydroxyl ions (OH^-) than hydrogen ions (H^+). A pH greater than 7. Also called a *basic solution*.

Alkalosis   A condition in which blood pH is higher than 7.45. Also called *alkalemia*.

Amino acid   An organic acid that contains an acid carboxyl group (–COOH) and a basic amino group ($-NH_2$). Amino acids are building blocks from which proteins are formed.

Amino group $-NH_2$.

Ammonia NH_3.

Ammonium ion NH_4^+.

Anal triangle   The subdivision of the female or male perineum that contains the anus. (The perineum is a diamond-shaped area between the thighs and buttocks.)

Angiotensin   Either of two forms of a protein that is involved in the regulation of blood pressure.

Angiotensin I   A protein that results from the action of renin on angiotensinogen (a plasma protein). It is converted into angiotensin II by the action of angiotensin converting enzyme (ACE).

Angiotensin II   A hormone produced by the action of angiotensin converting enzyme (ACE) on angiotensin I. It stimulates aldosterone secretion by the adrenal cortex and the release of ADH by the posterior pituitary gland. It acts on arterioles, causing vasoconstriction; and acts on the thirst center in the hypothalamus, stimulating thirst. All of these actions tend to raise the arterial blood pressure.

Angiotensin converting enzyme (ACE)   An enzyme that converts angiotensin I into angiotensin II. It is abundant in the endothelial cells lining the capillaries of the lungs.

Angiotensinogen   A plasma protein produced by the liver. The enzyme renin converts angiotensinogen into angiotensin I.

Anion   A negatively charged ion. An example is the chloride ion (Cl^-).

ANP   *See* Atrial natriuretic peptide.

ANS   *See* Autonomic nervous system.

Antidiuretic   A substance that inhibits urine formation.

Antidiuretic hormone (ADH)   A hormone that decreases urine production (diuresis). It is secreted by the hypothalamus and released into the bloodstream by the posterior pituitary gland. It causes water retention by acting on the principal cells lining the collecting ducts of the kidneys, causing them to be more permeable to water. It also causes vasoconstriction of arterioles. Both actions tend to raise the arterial blood pressure. Also called *vasopressin*.

Antiport   A type of secondary active transport. A process by which two substances, usually sodium (Na^+) and another substance, move in opposite directions across a plasma membrane. In most cells, Na^+/Ca^{2+} antiports keep Ca^{2+} concentration low in the cytosol. Na^+/H^+ antiports help regulate the cytosol's pH by using the Na^+ gradient to expel H^+. Also called *countertransport*.

Antiporter   An integral membrane protein that acts as a carrier in an antiport. These proteins have two binding sites, one for sodium ions and one for the actively transported solute. Also called a *countertransporter*.

Anuria   A daily urine output of less than 50 ml. Anuria occurs when the blood hydrostatic pressure in the glomeruli falls

115

to 42 mmHg, causing filtration to stop.

Apical membrane   The portion of the membrane of an epithelial cell that is in direct contact with the filtrate in the lumen of a renal tubule. Also called the *luminal membrane*.

Arcuate arteries   In the kidney, branches of the interlobar arteries that arch between the medulla and the cortex.

Arcuate veins   In the kidney, veins that drain the interlobar veins. They arch between the medulla and the cortex.

Areolar connective tissue   A type of loose connective tissue that immediately underlies the epithelial lining of the urinary bladder.

Arteriole   A small, almost microscopic, artery that delivers blood to a capillary.

Ascending limb of the loop of Henle   The second portion of the loop of Henle. It carries filtrate from a U-shaped bend in the medulla upward to the cortex.

ATP   *See* Adenosine triphosphate.

Atrial natriuretic peptide (ANP)   A hormone secreted by cells in the atria of the heart in response to stretching. It promotes the excretion of water (diuresis) and the excretion of sodium (natriuresis).

Autonomic nervous system (ANS)   One of the two major subdivisions of the peripheral nervous system. Its sensory (afferent) neurons conduct impulses to the central nervous system (CNS) from visceral organs (internal organs). Its motor (efferent) neurons conduct impulses from the CNS to smooth muscle, cardiac muscle, and glands. The ANS is divided into sympathetic and parasympathetic divisions.

Autonomic plexus   An extensive network of sympathetic and parasympathetic nerve fibers. The cardiac, celiac, and pelvic plexuses are located in the thorax, abdomen, and pelvis, respectively.

Autoregulation   A local, automatic adjustment of blood flow in a given region of the body in response to tissue needs.

Balance concept   To maintain a relatively constant level of a substance in the body, the amount ingested and produced must equal the amount excreted and consumed.

Baroreceptor   A receptor that is sensitive to changes in pressure. Also called a *pressoreceptor*.

Base   A proton acceptor, or a nonacid; characterized by an excess of hydroxyl ions (OH⁻) and a pH greater than 7.

Basement membrane   A layer of extracellular material that attaches epithelial tissue to the underlying connective tissue; consists of the basal lamina and reticular lamina. The basement membrane of the glomerulus lies between the endothelium (of the capillaries) and the epithelium (of the visceral layer of the glomerular capsule).

Basolateral membrane   The portion of the membrane of an epithelial cell that is in contact with the interstitial fluid surrounding a renal tubule. The membrane enclosing the base and sides of the cell.

Basic solution   *See* Alkaline solution.

BCOP   *See* Blood colloid osmotic pressure.

Benzoic acid   A toxic substance found in fruits and vegetables. Converted into hippuric acid by liver cells and excreted.

Bicarbonate ion   HCO₃⁻.

Bile   A secretion of the liver that is stored in the gallbladder. Consists of water, bile salts, bile pigments, cholesterol, lecithin, and several ions. It causes the dispersion of large fat droplets into smaller fat droplets (emulsification).

Bilirubin   A red pigment that is one of the end products of hemoglobin breakdown in the liver cells; it is excreted as a waste material in the bile.

Bilirubinuria   The presence of above–normal levels of bilirubin in urine.

Biliverdin   A green pigment that is one of the first products of hemoglobin breakdown in liver cells; it is converted into bilirubin and excreted as a waste material in bile.

Blood colloid osmotic pressure (BCOP)   In the kidney, one of two forces that oppose filtration. It is the osmotic pressure that is due to the presence of proteins in blood plasma (and the absence of proteins in the filtrate). As a result of BCOP, water tends to move out of the filtrate and back into blood of the glomerular capillary. BCOP equals about 27 mm Hg.

Blood plasma   *See* Plasma.

Blood urea nitrogen (BUN)   A screening test that can provide information about kidney function. It measures the nitrogen in blood that is present in molecules of urea.

Body compartments   *See* Fluid compartments.

Body fluid   Body water and its dissolved substances.

Bowman's capsule   *See* Glomerular capsule.

Bowman's space   *See* Capsular space.

Brush border   The fuzzy line that is seen in a photomicrograph of the intestinal lining (taken through a light microscope). It is caused by the microvilli (fingerlike projections) on the apical (free) surface of the absorptive epithelial cells.

Buffer system   A pair of chemicals, one a weak acid and one the salt of the weak acid, which functions as a weak base. Buffer systems resist changes in the pH.

Bulk transport   A mechanism for moving substances across plasma membranes that requires the energy derived from splitting ATP. Bulk transport moves large particles, such as bacteria, blood cells, polysaccharides, and proteins. There are two general types of bulk transport: endocytosis moves particles into cells and exocytosis moves particles out of cells. *Also see* Endocytosis and Exocytosis.

BUN   *See* Blood urea nitrogen.

Ca   *See* Calcium.

Ca²⁺   *See* Calcium ion.

CA   *See* Carbonic anhydrase.

Caffeine   A substance that stimulates urine excretion (diuresis). In the kidney, it inhibits sodium reabsorption; therefore, inhibits water reabsorption.

Calcitonin   A hormone produced by the thyroid gland. It lowers the calcium and phosphate levels of the blood by inhibiting bone breakdown and accelerating calcium uptake by the bones.

Calcitriol   A hormone synthesized and secreted by the kidneys and produced in the skin by ultraviolet light. Its actions increase the levels of calcium and phosphorus in the blood. It stimulates the absorption of dietary calcium and phosphorus in the intestine and the reabsorption of calcium by the kidneys. Also called *1, 25–dihydroxycholecalciferol* and *1, 25–dihydroxy vitamin D*.

Calcium (Ca)   A bulk mineral. Important for bone development, nerve and muscle function, and blood clotting.

Calcium ion (Ca²⁺)   The most abundant ion in the body. A large amount is stored in bones.

Calculi   *See* Calculus.

Calculus (plural: calculi)   A stone or insoluble mass of crystallized salt or other material. Calculi are formed in the gallbladder, kidney, or urinary bladder.

Calyses (singular: calyx) *See* Calyx.

Calyx (plural: calyses) A cuplike division of the renal pelvis.

Candida albicans The most common fungus to appear in urine. A cause of vaginitis.

Capsular hydrostatic pressure (CHP) In the kidney, one of two forces that oppose filtration. CHP tends to push filtrate back into the glomerular capillary. It equals about 15 mm Hg.

Capsular space The space between the parietal and visceral layers of the glomerular (Bowman's) capsule. Also called *Bowman's space.*

Carbon dioxide CO_2.

Carbonic acid H_2CO_3.

Carbonic acid-bicarbonate buffer system The most abundant buffer system in the extracellular fluid (ECF).

Carbonic anhydrase (CA) An enzyme that causes carbon dioxide to combine with water to form carbonic acid. It is present in red blood cells and in epithelial cells lining certain portions of the renal tubules.

Carboxyl group —COOH.

Carotid body chemoreceptor A receptor (nerve ending) on or near the carotid sinus that responds to changes in blood levels of oxygen, carbon dioxide, and hydrogen ions.

Carotid sinus A dilated region of the internal carotid artery located just above the bifurcation of the common carotid artery. Contains sensory nerve endings (baroreceptors) that monitor blood pressure.

Carotid sinus baroreceptor A receptor (nerve ending) in the carotid sinus that responds to stretch or distortion produced by changes in arterial blood pressure.

Cast A small mass of hardened material formed within a cavity in the body and then discharged from the body. Casts are present in the urine.

Catheter A flexible tube that can be inserted into a body channel, such as a vein or the urethra, to distend or maintain an opening.

Catheterization The insertion of a catheter. The insertion of a catheter through the urethra into the urinary bladder permits urine to flow freely.

Cation A positive ion. Example: a sodium ion (Na^+).

Cerebrospinal fluid (CSF) A fluid produced by the choroid plexuses, which are located in the four ventricles of the brain. It circulates in the ventricles of the brain and in the subarachnoid space surrounding the brain and spinal cord.

Chemical element A unit of matter that cannot be decomposed into a simpler substance by ordinary chemical reactions. Examples include hydrogen (H), carbon (C), and oxygen (O). There are approximately 100 elements.

Chemical gradient *See* Concentration gradient.

Chloride ion (Cl^-) The major extracellular anion.

Chlorine (Cl) A bulk mineral. Important for acid-base balance, water balance, and the formation of hydrochloric acid (HCl).

CHP *See* Capsular hydrostatic pressure.

Cl *See* Chlorine.

Cl$^-$ *See* Chloride ion.

Clearance *See* Renal plasma clearance.

CO_2 Carbon dioxide.

Collecting duct A collecting duct links a distal convoluted tubule (DCT) to a papillary duct, which drains into a minor calyx of the renal pelvis. In collecting ducts, the reabsorption of sodium is controlled by aldosterone; the reabsorption of

water is controlled by antidiuretic hormone (ADH). The secretion of hydrogen and potassium ions occurs in this portion of the renal tubule.

Colloid A large molecule that cannot pass through capillary walls. Usually a protein.

Compensation The physiological response to an acid–base imbalance. There are two types: respiratory compensation(fast, occurs within minutes) and metabolic compensation (slow, takes days).

Concentration The amount of substance (solute) per unit volume of solution.

Concentration gradient The difference in concentration between two areas. If a particular ion or molecule is present in high concentration in one area and in low concentration in another area, the difference in concentration is called the concentration gradient. There is a net diffusion of particles from an area of high to low concentration; *down* or *with* the concentration gradient. Also called a *chemical gradient*.

Convoluted Convoluted tubules mean coiled tubules (rather than straight).

—COOH Carboxyl group.

Coronal plane *See* Frontal plane.

Cortex An outer layer of any organ.

Cortical nephron One of the two types of nephrons. Its renal corpuscle (glomerulus and glomerular capsule) is located in the outer portion of the cortex. It has a short loop of Henle. About 80% of all nephrons are of this type. Also called a *short-loop nephron*.

Cotransport *See* Symport.

Cotransporter *See* Symporter.

Countercurrent exchanger system A mechanism that depends upon the countercurrent flow of blood in the vasa recta of juxtamedullary nephrons. It maintains the interstitial osmolarity that is generated by the countercurrent multiplier system (loop of Henle).

Countercurrent flow Fluid flowing in opposite directions in two nearby tubes. In the kidney, this occurs with the loop of Henle and the vasa recta (capillaries) of juxtamedullary nephrons; in both cases there is a descending and an ascending portion, forming a hairpin loop.

Countercurrent mechanism A mechanism involved in the production of concentrated (hyperosmotic) urine. It is dependent upon the anatomical arrangement of the loops of Henle (countercurrent multiplier system) and the vasa recta (countercurrent exchanger system).

Countercurrent multiplier system A mechanism that depends upon the countercurrent flow of filtrate in the loop of Henle. It generates an osmotic gradient in the medullary interstitium.

Countertransport *See* Antiport.

Countertransporter *See* Antiporter.

Creatinine A waste product derived primarily from the breakdown of creatine phosphate (nitrogenous substance in muscle tissue). It is present in urine.

CSF *See* Cerebrospinal fluid.

DCT *See* Distal convoluted tubule.

Deamination Removal of an amino group ($-NH_2$) from an amino acid, forming a keto acid (a type of carbohydrate).

Deciliter (dl) 0.1 liter.

Dehydration Excessive loss of water from the body or its parts. When water loss is greater than water gain. Also called *hypovolemia*.

Descending limb of the loop of Henle   The first portion of the loop of Henle. It carries filtrate down into the medulla.

Detrusor muscle   A muscle layer surrounding the mucosa of the urinary bladder. It consists of three layers of smooth muscle, which contract in response to parasympathetic stimulation.

Diabetes insipidus   A condition caused by hyposecretion of antidiuretic hormone (ADH). It is characterized by thirst and excretion of large amounts of dilute urine.

Diabetes mellitus   A hereditary condtion caused by hyposecretion of insulin. It is characterized by excessive eating, excessive thirst, increased urine production, and hyperglycemia (above normal blood glucose levels).

Dialysate   The molecules that pass through the dialyzing membrane during dialysis.

Dialysis   The process of separating molecules by the difference in their rates of diffusion through a selectively permeable membrane. Crystalloids (small, noncolloids) pass through readily; colloids (large molecules) pass through very slowly or not at all.

Diffusion   A passive process in which there is a net movement of molecules or ions from a region of high concentration to a region of low concentration until equilibrium is reached. Also called *simple diffusion* (as opposed to facilitated diffusion).

1, 25 – dihydroxycholecalciferol   *See* Calcitriol.

1, 25 – dihydroxy vitamin D₃   *See* Calcitriol.

Distal   Farther from the point of origin. For example, the distal convoluted tubule is farther from the renal corpuscle than the proximal convoluted tubule.

Distal convoluted tubule (DCT)   The portion of the renal tubule that is farther away from the renal corpuscle; located betweeen the loop of Henle and the collecting duct.

Diuresis   Increased urine excretion.

Diuretic   A drug that increases urine excretion. Caffeine inhibits sodium and water reabsorption; alcohol inhibits antidiuretic hormone (ADH) secretion. Both are diuretics.

dl   *See* Deciliter.

Dorsal   Nearer to the back; opposite of ventral. Also called *posterior*.

ECF   *See* Extracellular fluid.

Efferent   Carrying away from. Applies to blood vessels and nerves.

Efferent arteriole   In the kidney, a blood vessel that carries blood away from a glomerulus. It branches, forming peritubular capillaries.

Electric gradient   The difference in electrical charge between two areas.

Electric force   A force that causes charged particles to move away from a region having a like charge toward a region having the opposite charge.

Electrochemical gradient   A combined electrical and chemical gradient, such as exists across a plasma membrane.

Electrolyte   Any compound that separates into ions when dissolved in water.

Endocytosis   A mechanism for moving large particles into cells. It requires the energy derived from splitting ATP. A segment of the plasma membrane surrounds the substance to be taken in, encloses it, and brings it into the cell. There are three types of endocytosis: phagocytosis, pinocytosis,

and receptor-mediated endocytosis. *Also see* Phagocytosis, Pinocytosis, and Receptor-mediated endocytosis.

Endothelial-capsular membrane   The membrane that filters blood as it passes from the glomerular capillaries into the renal tubules. It consists of three layers: the endothelium of the glomerular capillaries; the epithelium of the visceral layer of the glomerular capsule; and the basement membrane between the endothelium and the epithelium.

Endothelium   A type of epithelial tissue. It lines blood vessels, lymphatic vessels, and the cavities of the heart.

Enuresis   Involuntary discharge of urine, complete or partial, after age three. *Also see* Incontinence.

Enzyme   A substance that affects the speed of a specific chemical reaction; an organic catalyst, usually a protein.

Epithelial tissue   One of the four basic types of tissues. It includes covering epithelium, lining epithelium, and glandular epithelium.

Erythropoiesis   The process by which red blood cells (erythrocytes) are formed.

Erythropoietin   A hormone secreted by the kidneys that stimulates the production of red blood cells.

Excretion   The process of eliminating waste products from a cell, tissue, or the entire body; or the products excreted.

Exocytosis   A mechanism for moving large particles out of cells. It requires the energy derived from splitting ATP. Membrane-enclosed structures called secretory vesicles fuse with the plasma membrane and release their contents into the extracellular fluid. Protein hormones and digestive enzymes are released from secretory cells in this way.

External urethral orifice   The opening of the urethra to the exterior.

External urethral sphincter   A sphincter (valve) that controls the flow of urine out of the urinary bladder. It consists of skeletal muscle and is under voluntary control.

Extracellular fluid (ECF)   One of the two major fluid compartments of the body. It includes blood plasma and interstitial fluid.

Facilitated diffusion   Diffusion in which a substance not soluble by itself in lipids is transported across a selectively permeable membrane by combining with a transporter (carrier molecule). Transporters are integral proteins in the plasma membrane. The most important substance that enters many body cells by facilitated diffusion is glucose. After glucose attaches to the transporter on the outside of the membrane, the transporter changes shape; glucose passes through the membrane and is released inside the cell.

Feces   Material discharged from the rectum; consists of bacteria, excretions, and food residue. Also called *stool*.

Feedback loop   *See* Feedback system.

Feedback system   A sequence of events in which information about the status of a situation is continually reported (fed back) to a central control region. Also called a *feedback loop* or *reflex arc*.

Fenestration   "Little window." Capillaries in which the endothelial cells appear to be perforated are called fenestrated capillaries.

Filtrate   The fluid produced when blood is filtered by the endothelial-capsular membrane. The endothelial-capsular membrane separates the blood in the glomerular capillaries from the filtrate in the capsular space of the glomerular capsule. Also called a *nephric filtrate* or *tubular fluid*.

Filtration   The passage of a liquid through a filter or a membrane that acts like a filter. Such movement is always from an area of higher pressure to an area of lower pressure; in the body the driving pressure is usually blood pressure. Most small to medium-sized molecules such as nutrients, gases, ions, hormones, and vitamins can be forced through cell membranes, but large proteins cannot.

Filtration fraction   In the kidneys, the percentage of plasma entering the nephrons that becomes glomerular filtrate.

Filtration slit   In the kidney, filtration slits are spaces between the pedicels (feet) of podocytes (specialized epithelial cells that form the visceral layer of the glomerular capsule). Also called a *slit pore*.

Fixed acid   An acid that cannot be eliminated by exhalation. Also called *nonvolatile acid*.

Fluid balance   Fluid balance means water balance. The required amount of water is present in the appropriate proportions in the fluid compartments of the body.

Fluid compartments   The three basic fluid compartments in the body: intracellular fluid (ICF), extracellular fluid (ECF), and plasma. Also called *body compartments*.

Fluid intake   Daily water gain; about 2500 ml/day.

Fluid output   Daily water loss; about 2500 ml/day. Fluid loss is regulated by three hormones: antidiuretic hormone (ADH), aldosterone, and atrial natriuretic hormone (ANP).

Frontal plane   A plane that runs vertical to the ground and divides the body into anterior and posterior portions. It is at right angles to the sagittal plane. Also called the *coronal plane*.

Gastrointestinal tract   A continuous tube running through the ventral body cavity extending from the mouth to the anus. Also called the *GI tract* or the *alimentary canal*.

GBHP   *See* Glomerular blood hydrostatic pressure.

GI tract   *See* Gastrointestinal tract.

Glomerular blood hydrostatic pressure (GBHP)   The blood pressure in the glomerular capillaries. Equal to about 60 mm Hg.

Glomerular capsule   One of the two components of a renal corpuscle (the other component is a glomerulus). It is a double-walled cup, consisting of epithelial cells, which surrounds a glomerulus (tuft of capillary loops). Also called *Bowman's capsule*.

Glomerular filtration   The first step in the production of urine. Blood pressure forces water and dissolved blood components through the endothelial–capsular membrane, forming the filtrate.

Glomerular filtration rate (GFR)   The amount of filtrate that forms in all the renal corpuscles of both kidneys each minute. In the normal adult, the GFR is about 125 ml/min. This amounts to about 180 liters (48 gal.) each day.

Glomerulus   One of the two components of a renal corpuscle (the other component is a glomerular capsule). It consists of a tuft of capillary loops. Blood enters a glomerulus via an afferent arteriole and exits via an efferent arteriole.

Gluconeogenesis   The conversion of a substance other than carbohydrate into glucose. Gluconeogenesis occurs in the kidneys during periods of fasting or starvation.

Glucose   A six-carbon sugar, $C_6H_{12}O_6$. The major energy source for every cell type in the body.

Glucosuria   *See* Glycosuria.

Glycosuria   The presence of glucose in the urine. Also called *glucosuria*.

Gradient   A gradual increase or decrease of a variable over distance. Examples are pressure gradients, electrical gradients, and concentration gradients.

Granular cells   *See* Juxtaglomerular cells.

H   Hydrogen.

H$^+$ Hydrogen ion.

HCl   Hydrochloric acid.

HCO$_3^-$ Bicarbonate ion.

H$_2$CO$_3$ Carbonic acid.

Hematuria   Blood in the urine.

Hemodialysis   Cleansing of the blood by dialysis.

Hilum   *See* Hilus.

Hilus   A notch near the center of the concave border of a kidney. At this location, the ureter leaves the kidney. Blood vessels, lymphatic vessels, and nerves enter and exit the kidney through the hilus. Also called *hilum*.

Hippuric acid   The form in which benzoic acid (a toxic substance in fruits and vegetables) is excreted in urine.

Histology   Microscopic study of tissues.

Homeostasis   The relative stability of the internal environment (extracellular fluid). It results from the actions of feedback systems (reflex arcs or feedback loops), which constantly monitor changes and make adjustments by negative feedback.

HPO$_4^{2-}$ Phosphate.

Hydro   The Greek work meaning water.

Hydrochloric acid   HCl.

Hydrogen   H.

Hydrogen ion   H$^+$.

Hydrostatic pressure   The force that a fluid under pressure exerts against the walls of its container.

Hydroxyl group   –OH.

Hyper –   Too much.

Hypercalcemia   Abnormally high plasma calcium.

Hyperkalemia   Abnormally high plasma potassium.

Hypermagnesemia   Abnormally high plasma magnesium.

Hypernatremia   Abnormally high plasma sodium.

Hyperosmotic solution   *See* Hypertonic solution.

Hyperphosphatemia   Abnormally high plasma phosphate.

Hypertonic solution   A solution that has a higher concentration of solutes and a lower concentration of water than the intracellular fluid inside cells. Water moves by osmosis out of the cell (down its concentration gradient). Also called a *hyperosmotic solution*.

Hypervolemia   See Water intoxication.

Hypo –   Too little.

Hypocalcemia   Abnormally low plasma calcium.

Hypochloremia   Abnormally low plasma chloride.

Hypokalemia   Abnormally low plasma potassium.

Hypomagnesemia   Abnormally low plasma magnesium.

Hyponatremia   Abnormally low plasma sodium.

Hypo-osmotic solution   *See* Hypotonic solution.

Hyposmotic solution   *See* Hypotonic solution.

Hypophosphatemia   Abnormally low plasma phosphate.

Hypotonic solution   A solution that has a total solute concentration less than that of plasma. Also called a *hypo-osmotic solution* or *hyposmotic solution*.

Hypovolemia   *See* Dehydration.

Incontinence   Inability to retain urine, semen, or feces. Caused by loss of sphincter control.

Indican   Substance present in urine; potassium salt of indole.

Indole   A toxic by-product of protein catabolism. It is converted into indican in the liver.

Inorganic compound   One of the two main types of chemical compounds. Inorganic compounds usually lack carbon; usually are small and contain ionic bonds. Examples include water and many acids, bases, and salts.

Integral membrane protein   A protein embedded in the phospholipid bilayer of plasma membranes; may span the entire membrane or be located on just one side.

Intercalated cell   Cells located in the distal convoluted tubules and collecting ducts scattered among the more abundant principal cells. Intercalated cells can secrete hydrogen ions when the plasma pH levels are below normal.

Interlobar arteries   Interlobar arteries are branches of segmental arteries; they pass between the renal pyramids.

Interlobar veins   Interlobar veins drain arcuate veins and empty into segmental veins.

Interlobular arteries   Interlobular arteries are branches of arcuate arteries; they enter the cortex and divide, forming afferent arterioles.

Interlobular veins   Interlobular veins drain peritubular venules and empty into arcuate veins.

Internal urethral orifice   The internal urethral orifice is the opening to the urethra; it is located in the anterior corner of the trigone in the urinary bladder.

Internal urethral sphincter   A sphincter (valve) that controls the flow of urine out of the urinary bladder. It consists of smooth muscle fibers (detrusor muscle); parasympathetic stimulation causes the muscle to relax and the valve to open.

Interstitial fluid   The fluid in the interstitial spaces (between the cells). About 80% of the extracellular fluid (ECF).

Interstitium   The fluid-filled space between tissue cells.

Intracellular fluid (ICF)   The fluid inside the body cells. About 2/3 of the total body fluid.

Inulin   A polysaccharide that can be used to determine the glomerular filtration rate (GFR). Since it is not reabsorbed or secreted, inulin clearance equals the GFR, normally about 125 ml/min.

Ion   Any charged particle or group of particles; usually formed when a substance, such as a salt, dissolves and dissociates.

Ion channel   A water-filled channel formed by integral proteins in a plasma membrane. Small substances that are not lipid-soluble may diffuse into or out of a cell through an ion channel. Ions that pass through plasma membranes via ion channels include sodium ions (Na^+), potassium ions (K^+), calcium ions (Ca^{2+}), chloride ions (Cl^-), and bicarbonate ions (HCO_3^-). Also called a *leakage channel*.

Iso–osmotic solution   *See* Isotonic solution.

Isotonic saline   A 0.9% NaCl (salt) solution. Under normal cicumstances this solution is isosmotic (isotonic) to red blood cells (RBCs).

Isotonic solution   A solution that contains the same concentration of water molecules and impermeable solute particles as the intracellular fluid of cells. Also called an *iso-osmotic solution*.

JGA   *See* Juxtaglomerular apparatus.

JG cells   *See* Juxtaglomerular cells.

Juxta –   A prefix meaning located near or adjoining.

Juxtaglomerular apparatus (JGA)   A structure near the glomerulus. It consists of the macula densa and the juxtaglomerular cells. It is involved in the regulation of blood pressure and the glomerular filtration rate (GFR). The juxtaglomerular cells secrete renin, which initiates the renin–angiotensin pathway.

Juxtaglomerular cells (JG cells)   Modified smooth muscle cells in the wall of the afferent arteriole. Its granules contain renin. Also called *granular cells*.

Juxtamedullary nephron   A nephron with its renal corpuscle deep in the cortex close to the medulla. It has a long loop of Henle, and is important in the control of urine concentration. About 20% of the nephrons are of this type. Also called a *long–loop nephron*.

K   Potassium.

K$^+$ Potassium ion.

Ketones   *See* Ketone bodies.

Ketone bodies   Substances (acetone, acetoacetic acid, and beta-hydroxybutyric acid) produced during excessive triglyceride catabolism. Also called *ketones*.

Ketosis   Abnormal condition marked by excessive production of ketone bodies. Also called *acetonuria*.

Kidney   One of the paired reddish organs located in the lumbar region that regulates the composition and volume of blood and produces urine.

Kidney stones   Crystals of salts present in urine that have solidified, forming insoluble stones. They may be formed in any portion of the urinary tract. Also called *renal calculi*.

Lamina propria   The connective tissue layer of a mucous membrane. It underlies the transitional epithelium that lines the urinary bladder.

Leakage channel   *See* Ion channel.

Littre glands   *See* Urethral glands.

Long–loop nephron   *See* Juxtamedullary nephrons.

Loop of Henle   The portion of the renal tubule between the proximal convoluted tubule (PCT) and the distal convoluted tubule (DCT). It descends into the medulla, makes a hairpin turn, then returns upward to the cortex. Also called the *nephron loop*.

Lumen   The space within an artery, vein, intestine, or a tube.

Luminal membrane   *See* Apical membrane.

Macula densa   Part of the juxtaglomerular apparatus. It consists of cells of the distal convoluted tubule adjacent to the afferent and efferent arterioles (near the glomerulus).

Magnesium (Mg)   A bulk mineral. Important for bone development, nerve and muscle function, and a constituent of coenzymes.

Magnesium ion (Mg^{2+})   The second most abundant cation in the intracellular fluid (ICF).

Medulla   The innermost portion of an organ.

Medullary interstitium   In the kidney, the fluid in the interstitial spaces of the medulla. It is significant because it plays an important role in the process that concentrates urine. From the cortex to the renal pelvis, the medullary interstitium becomes progressively more concentrated.

Medullary pyramid   *See* Renal pyramid.

Membrane transport mechanisms   Mechanisms that move

substances across a plasma membrane (between the interstitial and intracellular fluids). There are two basic types: (1) active processes, which require energy from the splitting of ATP; (2) passive processes, which do not require energy from the splitting of ATP.

Membranous urethra   The portion of the urethra that passes through the urogenital diaphragm; between the prostatic urethra and the spongy urethra.

mEq/L   *See* Milliequivalents per liter.

Metabolic acidosis   Acidosis due to any cause other than accumulation of carbon dioxide; a bicarbonate (HCO_3^-) concentration below 22 mEq/liter.

Metabolic alkalosis   Alkalosis due to any cause other than excessive respiratory removal of carbon dioxide; a bicarbonate (HCO_3^-) concentration above 26 mEq/liter.

Metabolic water   The water produced during anabolic reactions (dehydration synthesis). It amounts to about 200 ml/day.

Metabolism   The sum of all the biochemical reactions that occur within an organism. Includes the synthetic (anabolic) reactions and decomposition (catabolic) reactions. The kidney has several metabolic functions, including glucose synthesis (gluconeogenesis), vitamin D activation (formation of calciferol), and red blood cell production (secretion of erythropoietin).

Metabolite   Any substance produced by metabolism.

Mg   Magnesium.

Mg²⁺   Magnesium ion.

Micrometer (μm)   1/1,000 mm. A microscopic unit of length.

Microvilli (singular: microvillus)   Small fingerlike projections formed by the plasma membrane of an epithelial cell, which greatly increase the surface area of the cell. They are characteristic of the epithelial cells lining the proximal convoluted tubule (PCT) and the small intestine.

Micturition   The expulsion of urine from the urinary bladder. Also called *urination* or *voiding*.

Micturition reflex   The desire to urinate. Stretch receptors in the urinary bladder transmit sensory impulses to the micturition reflex center in the sacral region of the spinal cord; parasympathetic impulses from the spinal cord cause contraction of the detrusor muscle and relaxation of the internal urethral sphincter.

Milliequivalents per liter (mEq/L)   Concentration of a solution expressed as the total number of ions.

Millimeter (mm)   1/1,000 meter or 0.04 in. A unit of length.

Millimoles per liter (mM/L)   Concentration of a solution expressed as the molecular weight in milligrams.

Milliosmoles per liter (mOsm/L)   Concentration of a solution expressed as the total number of particles (molecules and ions).

Mineral   Inorganic, homogeneous solid substance that may perform a function vital to life. Examples include calcium, sodium, potassium, iron, phosphorus, and chlorine.

mm   *See* Millimeter.

mM/L   *See* Millimoles per liter.

mOsm/L   *See* Milliosmoles per liter.

Mucosa   *See* Mucous membrane.

Mucous membrane   A membrane that lines a body cavity that opens to the exterior. Also called the *mucosa*.

Na   *See* Sodium.

Na⁺   *See* Sodium ion.

Na⁺–glucose symport   The process by which sodium ions and glucose molecules are transported across a plasma membrane in the same direction by secondary active transport. Also called *Na⁺ – glucose cotransport*.

Na⁺–glucose symporter   An integral membrane protein that carries sodium ions and glucose molecules across a plasma membrane in the same direction by secondary active transport. Also called *Na⁺ – glucose cotransporter*.

Na⁺/H⁺ antiport   The process by which sodium and hydrogen ions are transported across a plasma membrane in opposite directions. Also called *Na⁺/H⁺ countertransport*.

Na⁺/H⁺ antiporter   An integral membrane protein that carries sodium and hydrogen ions across a plasma membrane in opposite directions. Also called *Na⁺/H⁺ countertransporter*.

Na⁺–K⁺ ATPase   *See* Sodium pump.

Na⁺–K⁺–2Cl⁻ symport   The process by which one sodium, one potassium, and two chloride ions are transported across a plasma membrane in the same direction by secondary active transport. Also called *Na⁺–K⁺–2Cl⁻ cotransport*.

Na⁺–K⁺–2Cl⁻ symporter   An integral membrane protein that carries one sodium, one potassium, and two chloride ions across a plasma membrane in the same direction by secondary active transport. Also called *Na⁺–K⁺–2Cl⁻ cotransporter*.

Na⁺/K⁺ pump   *See* Sodium pump.

Nanometer (nm)   1/1,000 micrometer (μm). A microscopic unit of length, formerly called a millimicron.

Negative feedback   The principal governing most control systems. A mechanism of response in which a stimulus initiates actions that reverse or reduce the stimulus.

Nephric filtrate   *See* Filtrate.

Nephrology   Scientific study of the kidney.

Nephron   The structural and functional unit of the kidney. Consists of the renal corpuscle (glomerulus and glomerular capsule), proximal convoluted tubule (PCT), loop of Henle, distal convoluted tubule (DCT), and the collecting duct.

Nephron loop   *See* Loop of Henle.

Nephrosis   Any disease of the kidney.

Net diffusion   The difference in diffusion between two regions having different concentrations. More particles diffuse from the region of high concentration to the region of low concentration than diffuse in the opposite direction.

Net filtration pressure (NFP)   The net pressure that promotes glomerular filtration. It is calculated by subtracting the forces that oppose filtration (capsular hydrostatic pressure and blood colloid osmotic pressure) from the glomerular blood hydrostatic pressure.

NFP   *See* Net filtration pressure.

—NH₂   Amino group.

NH₃   Ammonia.

NH₄⁺   Ammonium ion.

nm   *See* Nanometer.

Nonelectrolyte   Compound with covalent bonds. When dissolved in a liquid, it does not form ions.

Nonvolatile acid   *See* Fixed acid.

Organic compound   One of the two main types of chemical compounds. Organic compounds always contain carbon and hydrogen atoms and are held together by covalent bonds. Examples include carbohydrates, lipids, proteins, and nucleic acids (DNA and RNA).

Osmolarity   The solute concentration of a solution. The higher the osmolarity, the lower the water concentration.

Osmoreceptor   A nerve cell that responds to changes in the osmolarity (osmotic pressure) of the surrounding fluid. In response to high osmotic pressure (low water concentration), osmoreceptors in the hypothalamus cause the synthesis and release of antidiuretic hormone (ADH).

Osmosis   The net movement of water molecules through a selectively permeable membrane from an area of high water concentration to an area of lower water concentration until an equilibrium is reached.

Osmotic gradient   The difference in the osmotic pressures in two solutions separated by a membrane permeable to water. It determines the direction and rate of flow of water by osmosis.

Osmotic pressure   The pressure required to prevent the osmosis of pure water across a selectively permeable membrane into a solution containing solutes.

Overhydration   An increase in intracellular water concentration. It is particularly disruptive to nerve cell function.

PAH   *See* Para–aminohippuric acid.

Papillary duct   A large tube that drains urine from collecting ducts and empties into a minor calyx of the renal pelvis.

Para-aminohippuric acid (PAH)   A nontoxic substance that can be used to measure the renal plasma flow. The clearance of PAH is the same as the renal plasma flow.

Parasympathetic nervous system   One of the two subdivisions of the autonomic nervous system. It is primarily concerned with digestive, reproductive, and urinary functions.

Parenchyma   The functional tissue of an organ, as opposed to the tissue (called stroma) that forms its framework.

Parietal layer   In the nephron, the outer wall of the glomerular capsule. It is separated from the inner wall (visceral layer) by the capsular (Bowman's) space.

PCT   *See* Proximal convoluted tubule.

Pedicel   The footlike extension of a podocyte.

Pelvic diaphragm   A sheet of skeletal muscle that forms the floor of the pelvis. It helps to support the internal organs (viscera) of the abdominal and pelvic cavities.

Penis   The male organ of copulation and of urinary excretion.

Peptide   A chain of fewer than 50 amino acids.

Percent concentration   Concentration expressed as the amount of solute in solution. For example, 0.9% NaCl means that 0.9 g of NaCl are dissolved 100 ml of solution.

Peristalsis   Successive rhythmic contractions along the wall of a hollow muscular structure.

Peritoneal cavity   The potential space between the parietal peritoneum and the visceral peritoneum.

Peritoneum   The largest serous membrane of the body. Lines the abdominal cavity and covers the viscera (abdominal organs). The superior surface of the urinary bladder is covered by the peritoneum.

Peritubular capillaries   A network of capillaries that is closely associated with the renal tubule. Substances are reabsorbed from the filtrate into the blood of the peritubular capillaries; hydrogen ions, potassium ions, and drugs are secreted from the blood of the peritubular capillaries into the filtrate of the renal tubules.

Ph   A symbol for the concentration of hydrogen ions in a solution. The pH scale extends from 0 to 14. A pH of 7 indicates neutrality; values less than 7 indicate increasing acidity; values higher than 7 indicate increasing alkalinity.

Phagocytosis   "Cell eating." A type of bulk transport; requires energy derived from the splitting of ATP. The movement of solid particles through the plasma membrane. Pseudopods extend around the substance, enclose it, and bring it into the cell, forming a phagocytic vesicle.

Phosphate group $—PO_4^{2-}$.

Phosphate buffer system   An important regulator of pH inside cells (intracellular fluid). It is also present in urine.

Phosphate ion (HPO_4^{2-})   An ion whose concentration is highest in the intracellular fluid (ICF).

Phosphorus (P)   A bulk mineral. Functions: bone development, nerve and muscle function, buffer systems, enzyme component, and energy transfer (ATP).

Pinocytosis   "Cell drinking." A type of bulk transport; requires energy derived from the splitting of ATP. The movement of extracellular fluid droplets through the plasma membrane. Pseudopods extend around the fluid, enclose it, and bring it into the cell, forming a pinocytic vesicle.

Plasma   The fluid portion of blood. Also called *blood plasma*.

Plasma creatinine   Measurement of plasma creatinine is a test often used to evaluate kidney function. Creatinine is the end product of the catabolism of creatine phosphate (present in skeletal muscle).

Plasma proteins   Proteins confined to the blood plasma (not present in other tissues of the body). They are the key substances that determine the osmotic gradient between plasma and interstitial fluid. In the kidney, they are too large to pass through the filter (endothelial–capsular membrane). There are three main types: albumins, globulins, and fibrinogen.

Plexus   A network of nerves, veins, or lymphatic vessels.

$—PO_4^{2-}$ Phosphate group.

Podocyte   Specialized epithelial cells that form the visceral layer of the glomerular capsule. They have footlike extensions called pedicels.

Positive feedback   A feedback system in which the response enhances the original stimulus.

Posterior   *See* Dorsal.

Potassium (K)   A bulk mineral. Important for nerve and muscle function.

Potassium ion (K^+)   The most abundant cation in the intracellular fluid (ICF).

Preformed water   Water intake from ingested liquids and foods. It amounts to about 2300 ml/day. As opposed to metabolic water, which is derived from anabolic reactions.

Pressoreceptor   *See* Baroreceptor.

Primary active transport   One of two types of active transport (the other is secondary active transport). The energy derived from splitting ATP *directly* moves a substance across the plasma membrane. The most prevalent primary active transport pump is the sodium pump. It pumps sodium ions (Na^+) out of the cell against their concentration gradient, maintaining a low concentration of sodium ions inside the cell (in the cytosol). *Also see* Sodium pump.

Principal cells   Cells that line the distal convoluted tubule (DCT) and collecting duct of a nephron (in the kidney). Principal cells become permeable to water when acted upon by antidiuretic hormone (ADH), increasing the reabsorption of water. In the parathyroid glands, the cells that secrete

parathyroid hormone (PTH) are also called principal cells.

Prostate gland   A doughnut-shaped gland inferior to the urinary bladder that surrounds the superior portion of the male urethra and secretes a slightly acidic solution that contributes to sperm motility and viability.

Prostatic urethra   The portion of the urethra that passes through the prostate gland.

Protein   An organic compound consisting of carbon, hydrogen, oxygen, nitrogen, and sometimes sulfur and phosphorus. Made up of amino acids linked by peptide bonds.

Protein buffer system   The most abundant buffer system in the intracellular fluid (ICF) and blood plasma.

Proximal   Nearer to the point of origin.

Proximal convoluted tubule (PCT)   The portion of the renal tubule that is closest to the renal corpuscle.

Pyuria   The presence of white blood cells and other components of pus in the urine.

Reabsorption   *See* Tubular reabsorption.

Receptor-mediated endocytosis   A type of bulk transport; requires energy derived from the splitting of ATP. A highly selective process by which cells can take up specific molecules or particles. It involves the binding of a substance (ligand) to its specific receptor at the extracellular surface of the plasma membrane; the membrane folds inward, forming an endocytic vesicle.

Reflex arc   *See* Feedback system.

Renal   Pertaining to the kidney.

Renal arteries   Blood vessels that carry oxygenated blood from the abdominal aorta to the kidneys.

Renal autoregulation of GFR   The ability of the kidneys to maintain a constant blood pressure and GFR (glomerular filtration rate) despite changes in the systemic arterial pressure. It operates by negative feedback systems that involve the juxtaglomerular apparatus (JGA).

Renal calculi   *See* Kidney stones.

Renal capsule   The innermost of the three tissue layers that surround each kidney. It is continuous with the ureter.

Renal clearance   *See* Renal plasma clearance.

Renal column   Portions of the cortex of the kidney that extend between renal pyramids.

Renal corpuscle   One of the the two basic parts of a nephron. It has two components: the glomerulus and the glomerular capsule.

Renal fascia   The outermost layer of tissue surrounding each kidney. A thin layer of dense irregular connective tissue that anchors the kidney to its surrounding structures and to the abdominal wall.

Renal papilla   (plural: renal papillae)   The apex of a renal pyramid. Points toward the center of the kidney. The papillary duct passes through the renal papilla and empties into the renal pelvis.

Renal pelvis   A funnel-shaped cavity that is continuous with the ureter. The edge of the renal pelvis contains cuplike extensions called calyces.

Renal plasma clearance   A test for the evaluation of kidney function. It measures how effectively the kidneys remove (clear) a substance from blood plasma. Also called *renal clearance* or *clearance*.

Renal plexus   A network of nerves that supply the kidneys.

Renal pyramid   One of the 8 to 18 cone-shaped (pyramid-shaped) structures in each kidney that constitute the me-

dulla. Also called *medullary pyramid*.

Renal sinus   A cavity in the kidney. The renal pelvis is within the renal sinus.

Renal threshold   The plasma concentration at which a substance begins to spill into the urine.

Renal tubule   The tubular portion of a nephron. It consists of the proximal convoluted tubule (PCT), loop of Henle, distal convoluted tubule (DCT), and collecting duct.

Renal vein   A single vein that carries blood from each kidney to the inferior vena cava.

Renin   An enzyme secreted by the kidneys. It initiates the renin–angiotensin pathway, which increases the arterial blood pressure.

Renin-angiotensin pathway   A mechanism for the control of aldosterone secretion. In response to low blood pressure, renin is secreted by the kidneys; it causes the formation of angiotensin II, which stimulates the adrenal cortex to secrete aldosterone. Aldosterone increases the reabsorption of sodium (and water), increasing blood volume and blood pressure. Angiotensin II causes vasoconstriction of arterioles, raising the arterial blood pressure.

Respiratory acidosis   Acidosis due to excess carbon dioxide in the plasma. Carbon dioxide combines with water to form carbonic acid, which releases hydrogen ions (H^+).

Respiratory alkalosis   Alkalosis due to abnormally low concentrations of carbon dioxide in the plasma; the result is a decreased concentration of hydrogen ions (H^+).

Retention   A failure to completely or normally empty the bladder of urine.

Retroperitoneal organs   Organs located behind the peritoneum. The kidneys, pancreas, and some portions of the large intestine.

Rugae   (singular: ruga)   Large folds in the mucosa of an empty hollow organ, such as the stomach, urinary bladder, and vagina.

Secondary active transport   One of two types of active transport. The energy stored in ion gradients drives substances across the membrane. Since the ion gradients are established by primary active transport pumps, secondary active transport *indirectly* uses energy obtained from splitting ATP.

Secretion   *See* Tubular secretion.

Segmental arteries   Arteries that branch from the anterior and posterior branches of the renal artery.

Segmental veins   Veins that drain interlobar veins and empty into a single renal vein.

Selectively permeable membrane   A membrane that permits the passage of certain substances, but restricts the passage of others. A plasma membrane enclosing the cytoplasm of a cell is a selectively permeable membrane. Also called a *semipermeable membrane*.

Semipermeable membrane   *See* Selectively permeable membrane.

Serosa   A fibrous connective tissue that covers most of the bladder and is continuous with the same coat of the urethra. (The superior surface of the urinary bladder is covered by peritoneum.)

Serous membranes   Membranes that line a body cavity that does not open directly to the exterior, and cover the organs that lie within the cavity. They consist of thin layers of areolar connective tissue covered by a layer of mesothelium. They are composed of two portions: the parietal portion attached to the cavity wall and the visceral portion attached to the organs inside the cavities. Include the membranes that line the pleural, pericardial, and peritoneal cavities.

Short–loop nephron *See* Cortical nephron.

Slit membrane A thin membrane that extends across a filtration slit. (Filtration slits are the spaces between the footlike extensions of podocytes in renal corpuscles.)

Slit pore *See* Filtration slit.

Simple diffusion *See* Diffusion.

SO_4^{2-} Sulfate ion.

Sodium (Na) A bulk mineral. Important for nerve and muscle function, buffer systems, and electrolyte balance.

Sodium ion (Na^+) The most abundant ion in the extracellular fluid (ECF).

Sodium pump The most prevalent primary active transport pump. It maintains a low concentration of sodium ions in the cytosol by pumping them out against their concentration gradient. It also moves potassium ions into cells against their concentration gradient. Sodium and potassium ions constantly move through leakage channels (ion channels) down their concentration gradients, so sodium pumps must work constantly. All cells have hundreds of sodium pumps in each square micrometer of membrane surface. Also called *Na^+/K^+ ATP-ase* or *Na^+/K^+ pump*.

Solute A substance dissolved in a liquid.

Solution A mixture of one or more substances (solutes) dissolved in a liquid (solvent).

Solvent The liquid portion of a solution.

Specific gravity Density. The ratio of the weight of a substance to the weight of an equal volume of water. The specific gravity of urine ranges from 1.001 to 1.035.

Sphincter A ring of smooth muscle surrounding a tube. It functions as a valve; as the muscle contracts, the tube closes.

Spongy urethra The portion of the urethra that passes through the penis.

Starling's law of the capillaries A state of near equilibrium at the arterial and venous ends of a capillary. The quantity of fluid leaving the capillary at the arterial end nearly equals the quantity reabsorbed into the venous end. (Excess interstitial fluid is drained by the lymphatic system.)

Stool *See* Feces.

Strong acid When dissolved in water, a strong acid ionizes completely, forming hydrogen ions and the corresponding anions. A large quantity of hydrogen ions are released into solution. An example is hydrochloric acid (HCl).

Submucosa A layer of connective tissue located beneath a mucous membrane. The submucosa connects the mucous membrane (mucosa) to the muscularis layer.

Substrate A substance (metabolite) with which an enzyme reacts.

Sudoriferous glands A gland in the dermis or subcutaneous layer of the skin that produces perspiration. Also called a *sweat gland*.

Sulfate ion SO_4^{2-}

Sulfur A bulk mineral. Functions: hormone component; vitamin component; and ATP production.

Sweat gland *See* Sudoriferous gland.

Sympathetic nervous system One of the two subdivisions of the autonomic nervous system. It is primarily concerned with stress responses (fight–or-flight responses).

Symport A type of secondary active transport. A process by which two substances, usually Na^+ and another substance, move in the same direction across a cell membrane. Glucose, fructose, and amino acids enter cells lining the GI tract and the kidney tubules via symports. They return to the blood nutrients filtered by the kidneys so they are not lost in the urine. Also called *cotransport*.

Symporter An integral membrane protein that acts as a carrier in a symport. Also called *cotransporter*.

Tight junction A cell junction that is common in epithelial cells that line tubes. It prevents fluid from leaking from the lumen of a tube into the interstitial spaces.

T_m *See* Transport maximum.

Toxic materials Substances poisonous to the body.

Transitional epithelium Epithelium that is able to stretch. It lines organs such as the urinary bladder that continually inflate and deflate.

Transport maximum (T_m) The upper limit on how fast a given type of symport or antiport can operate. It is measured in mg/min.

Trichomonas vaginalis A protozoan (one-celled animal) that causes vaginitis in females and urethritis in males.

Trigone A small triangular area in the floor of the urinary bladder. Location of openings to the ureters and urethra.

Tubular fluid *See* Filtrate.

Tubular reabsorption The movement of water and solutes (especially nutrients) from the filtrate back into the blood in the peritubular capillaries. Most of the nutrients and water are reabsorbed in the first portion of the renal tubule, the proximal convoluted tubule (PCT). Also called *reabsorption*.

Tubular secretion One of the three main processes involved in urine formation. Substances from the blood in the peritubular capillaries are secreted into the filtrate. Substances secreted include hydrogen ions, potassium ions, ammonium ions, and certain drugs. Also called *secretion*.

Tubule A small tube.

Turbidity Cloudiness of a liquid. Urine is transparent when freshly voided; it becomes turbid upon standing.

Urea A nitrogenous waste derived from the deamination of amino acids. In the liver, ammonia, formed by deamination, combines with carbon dioxide to form urea. Urea constitutes 60–90% of all nitrogenous wastes in the urine.

Uremia A toxic level of urea in the blood.

Ureter A tube that extends from each kidney to the urinary bladder. Peristaltic contractions force urine down the ureters to the urinary bladder.

Urethra A small tube leading from the floor of the urinary bladder to the exterior of the body.

Urethral glands Glands in the spongy urethra of the male penis that produce mucus for lubrication during sexual intercourse. Also called *Littre glands*.

Urinalysis Analysis of urine.

Urinary bladder A hollow muscular organ located in the pelvic cavity, used to store and expel urine.

Urinary system Two kidneys, two ureters, one urinary

bladder, and one urethra.

Urination *See* Micturition.

Uric acid A nitrogenous waste derived from the catabolism of nucleic acids. Excessive uric acid crystallizes and deposits in joints, kidneys, and soft tissue; a condition known as gout.

Urine The fluid produced by the kidneys that contains wastes or excess materials and is excreted from the body through the urethra.

Urobilinogen A nitrogenous waste product of hemoglobin catabolism.

Urobilinogenuria The presence of urobilinogen in the urine.

Urology The branch of medicine that is concerned with the urinary tract in both males and females, and with the external reproductive organs (genitalia) in males.

Vasa recta Extensions of the efferent arteriole of a juxtamedullary nephron. Long, loop-shaped vessels that run parallel to the loop of Henle. They are important for the maintenance of the solute concentration in the medulla.

Vasopressin *See* Antidiuretic hormone.

Viscera (singular: viscus) The organs inside the body cavity.

Visceral Pertaining to the viscera.

Visceral layer In the nephron, the inner wall of the glomerular capsule. It is separated from the outer wall (parietal layer) by the capsular (Bowman's) space.

Visceral peritoneum Serous membrane that covers some of the viscera.

Voiding *See* Micturition.

Volatile acid An acid that can be eliminated by exhaling.

Water intoxication Excessive body fluid, causing electrolyte imbalance. Also called *hypervolemia*.

Weak acid When dissolved in water, weak acids do not completely ionize (some molecules do not dissociate). Consequently, fewer hydrogen ions are released into solution. An example is carbonic acid (H_2CO_3).

Bibliography

Curtis, Helena. *Biology,* 3rd ed.
New York : Worth, 1979.

Dorland, William Alexander. *Dorland's Illustrated Medical Dictionary,* 27th ed.
Philadelphia : W. B. Saunders, 1988.

Ganong, William F. *Review of Medical Physiology,* 15th ed.
Norwalk, Connecticut : Appleton & Lange, 1991.

Junqueira, L. Carlos, Jose Carneiro, and Robert O. Kelley. *Basic Histology*, 6th ed.
Norwalk, Connecticut : Appleton & Lange, 1989.

Kimball, John W. *Biology*, 4th ed.
Reading, Massachusetts : Addison-Wesley, 1978.

Melloni, B.J., Ida Dox, and Gilbert Eisner. *Melloni's Illustrated Medical Dictionary*, 2nd ed.
Baltimore : Williams & Wilkins, 1992.

Tortora, Gerard J. and Sandra Reynolds Grabowski. *Principles of Anatomy and Physiology,* 7th ed.
New York : HarperCollins, 1993.

Vander, Arthur J., James H. Sherman, and Dorothy S. Luciano. *Human Physiology,* 5th ed.
New York : McGraw-Hill, 1990.